The bad news: In the minute or two it takes to read this page, thirty people will die of easily preventable diseases as a result of poor lifestyle choices. These people weren't unintelligent, unmotivated, or unloved. What they were was overwhelmed. Most of them didn't have a daily health strategy of moving well, eating well, and thinking well, or they didn't bounce back when life's inevitable "mountains" got in the way.

The great news: The cure for health guilt, being overwhelmed, weight gain, low energy, poor sleep and disease is easy to understand and implement. The solutions you've been looking for are here in *Feet, Fork, and Fun: How to Fail Your Way to Fitness.*

Praise for *Feet, Fork, and Fun*

Dr. Tim, with personal stories and experiences, helps us each take 'baby steps' to transform our lives from victim to victor. If you want to live a more vibrant and fulfilling life, read Dr. Tim's book now.
    —Ken Keis, PhD., author of *The Quest For Purpose*

Dr. Warren gives the reader a unique perspective on health and fitness, one that is replete with insights based on both his professional background and also as an athlete. It's a no-nonsense, practical and holistic approach that is highly motivating.
    —Andre LeClair, PhD., Professor of Physics, Cornell University

This book will help many thousands easily adopt an active and vital lifestyle within their busy lives.
    —Sandra Musial, MD, Asistant Clinical Professor of Pediatrics, Brown University

Feet, Fork, and Fun *is not just another book on wellness. Dr. Tim Warren writes from years of experience as he holds our hand and shares with us the missing link that will lift us to that state of ultimate well being and optimum health.*
    —Rani St. Pucchi, Award winning fashion designer and best selling author of *The Soulmate Checklist* and *Your Body Your Style*

Quite an amazing guy who has written two really powerful books.
    —Jack Canfield, New York Times bestselling author of *The Success Principles* and co-author of the *Chicken Soup for the Soul* series

Very enjoyable and information-rich reading—truly worth while. Could be the difference that gets you to the summit.
    —Dennis Perman D.C.

Feet, Fork, and Fun

How to Fail Your Way to Fitness

by

Dr. Tim Warren

Dr. Tim Warren

Printed in the United States of America.

First Printing: January 2017

Wickford Press

wickfordpress.com

Feet, Fork, and Fun: How to Fail Your Way to Fitness is intended as a reference volume not as a medical manual. In light of individual, complex, and specific nature of health problems, this book is not intended to replace professional medical advice. The content, including ideas, procedures, and suggestions, in this book is intended to supplement, not replace, the advice of a trained medical professional. Consult him or her before adopting the suggestions in this book. The author and publisher disclaim any liability arising directly or indirectly from the use of this book.

Many of the designations used by manufacturers and sellers are claimed as trademarks. Where those designations appear in this book and the author and publisher were aware of the trademark claim, the designations have been printed with initial capital letters.

This book is available at quantity discounts for bulk purchases. For information call 401-374-5067.

Dedication

To Kelly, who makes me laugh every day.

Acknowledgments

Thanks to Steve Harrison and the crew of professionals at Bradley Communications for their help in the creation of this book, specifically: Steve himself, Rose, Deb, Geoffrey, Gail, and especially Martha Bullen, who took a special interest. Additional thanks to Laura Harrison for her insight and suggestions. The guru of graphics Alan Greco of Alan Greco Design has done awesome cover and interior design for both of my books. Special thanks to Heidi Grauel, editor, and Desiree Dugan for the professional photography, and doctors Dennis Perman and John Manning.

Contents

Why This Book Is for Losers 2

The Beta.. 7

Preface 9

Part One | Tone: Get It, Keep It... 12

Chapter One | One-Second Wellness...................................... 13

Chapter Two | Tone: The Mount Everest of Health 32

Chapter Three | Have a Nice Decay.. 45

Chapter Four | Feet, Fork, and Fun 60

Part Two | *Let's Roll*—Todd Beamer.. 71

Chapter Five | Feet: The Why of Moving Well 73

Chapter Six | Feet: The How of Moving Well 87

Chapter Seven | Fork: Eating Well.. 107

Chapter Eight | Fun: Thinking Well 118

Chapter Nine | Playing Twister with Your Great-Grandchildren..... 135

Chapter Ten | The Everest 70 Challenge 151

Appendix... 160

Why This Book Is for Losers

Are you one of the following fine, upstanding citizens?

- You are a hard worker putting in long days at work and paddling as fast as you can to keep yourself from being swept away. When you are not slaving away you are with your family trying your best to keep that ball successfully in the air. Too often the ball that gets dropped is fitness. The unhappy result is minimal exercise and a default to easy, quick processed food for you and your family. The only treadmill you are on is metaphorical.

- You are out of school, on your own, as smart as you will ever be, and ready to attack the world. But... you feel the grip of past failures in diet and exercise and you still have that extra thirty pounds and just can't seem to start on a "once and for all" health regimen.

- You have been a dedicated exerciser and have successfully instituted sweat into your life but you are dogged by low energy, poor sleep, and that pesky spare tire still bulges from under a race t-shirt.

- You are single and you painfully realize that your job has become your relationship. Your next thought is, "What happened to my body?"

- You have bought multiple exercise DVDs offered on late-night TV, have been on multiple diets, and bought every book you can get your hands on with not much to show for it except the satisfaction of doing your part to grease the economy.

- Are you a part-timer at work but a full-timer at home? You may have no time, no energy, and no hope of taking the time for yourself to get and stay fit. You wonder if this is as good as it gets and if you should just resign yourself to the status quo.

- Your kids are out or almost out of the house, retirement is in sight, but your body is racked with aches and pains and you wonder if there is any hope to feel good and have a healthy, fun, and meaningful retirement.

- You have a passionate desire to keep up and be a relevant force in your grandchildren's lives but you realize that without change it won't happen.

Do any of the above scenarios resonate? Perhaps you are a hybrid case with exhibited characteristics of several? Have you ever failed at fitness? Have you dropped the ball with an exercise program or a diet and are afraid to try again? This book is for you. Have you ever blown it and sabotaged an exercise program or a nutritional plan or both? Have you dropped the ball even when a diet or training regimen was working awesome? Have you felt guilty about blowing it? Have you felt down-right mad at your bad self? Have you been fed up and disgusted with the person in the mirror as a result? Have you silently called yourself a loser or a failure?

I'll make you a promise that you will never say any of these comments or think those thoughts again. However, you will mess up with fitness from time and time. I will and you will. It's not about blowing it, it's about picking up the pieces and getting going again... quickly. The secret to wellness is in shortening the time it takes to get back on the horse after you fall off. Fitness is all about a shortened reboot time.

This book is unlike any other health book or program. Sure, I will share unique and innovative strategies, powerful systems, and cutting-edge information for the reader to arrive at and remain at the top of your "mountain" with physical, chemical, and emotional well-being but the unique key is to forgive yourself, smack that reset button, and get back to healthy living. Sooner!

Let me ask you this, if you experience feelings of self-loathing does it inspire you to get back on the horse? Or do you do additional wallowing in the sewer of self-pity? I thought so. In fact, I know so because I have blown it a ton of times in my almost sixty years. Guess what? By the time you read this book and follow the step-by-step plan you will be in the best shape of your life and still be able to eat cake. By the way, you will still blow it occasionally. That's still cool. You may still fail and you may be mad at yourself, but now you will have the tools to mentally reboot quickly and decisively.

Dropping the fitness ball is not going to end with me or with you. The good news is it doesn't matter! The problem lies not in the failing but in not restarting sooner. We allow stinkin' thinkin' to persist when all we need is to get back on the yak. The solution is simply to reboot sooner. The secret to lifelong wellness is in shortening the reboot time and to keep putting one foot in front of the other. It's life and death but not complex. The secret is as simple as that. Cut down the reboot time, do more healthy stuff than unhealthy, and guess what? You win.

I have been bummed out, burned out, and pissed off at myself many times for failing at fitness. This from a guy who climbed the highest mountain on four continents, including Mount Everest at age forty-eight, ran his first twenty-six-mile marathon at age sixteen, counseled a quarter million patients on healthy living, and has never been more than a few ounces overweight in his entire life. More importantly, I watched as thousands of my patients failed time and time again at exercise or nutrition or both. I thought it was me. If I was a good doctor, then why couldn't I will my patients to better health? After all, they lined up to come see me. I changed my approach dozens of times thinking if I could just find the magic bullet then no one would fail again and my community and the world would be a healthier place.

After thirty years as a health care practitioner and caring for over 250,000 people and being a world class athlete myself, the truth gradually dawned on me that fitness failure was normal. It wasn't me and it wasn't really them. Dropping the ball in nutrition and exercise is a common human experience from top athletes to out-of-shape novices. Why do people fail at fitness? The world-shaking answer is that life gets in the way. It's called overwhelm. Yep, there is other stuff that is also important in today's world. I know this concept is shocking and hard to believe. My purpose is to present an innovative, easy, step-by-step, lifelong pathway to real health in three human dimensions without wasting a moment of your precious time.

Why should you listen to me about proper exercise, nutrition, and head space? First, I have injured myself many times from under-doing or overdoing exercise and I learned from all of it. Second, I have studied and experimented with many nutritional plans over the years. Many were good and many were, at best, worthless—and, at worst, dangerous. I became a vegetarian for four years before eating meat again. I devoured research. I joined more gyms than I could count, read more books than I could bench press, and hired trainers and coaches of all stripes. By far the most humbling but worthwhile education came after nine years of college, grad school, and multiple internships. The education that only comes from accepting the responsibility of caring for people. For thirty years, I was face-to-face with many dozens of people a day from CEOs to housewives to the homeless. Real people with real lives. People who wanted to be healthier naturally, without drugs. Some came as a first resort, some came as a last resort. They ranged from days old to 102 years old. I pleaded, cajoled, inspired, taught, mentored, demanded, exhorted, laughed, cried, and adjusted people to be healthier. From these years of experimenting with myself and constantly learning and caring for hundreds of patients per week I formulated the knowledge, building blocks, and principles that led me to the book you are holding in your hand right now. This book is for you.

Kim's Story

I was inspired to create this book by a woman who died decades ago. Kim was a thirty-something patient of mine whose family I cared for as a young doctor. Like myself and many of the folks I cared for at that time, she was a multitasking crazy person forcing her way through life. Two kids, job, husband, friends, home, and hobbies were all in the mix. Kim was decidedly not happy with herself. She was particularly vocal with me about her seeming inability to lose weight, exercise regularly, and feed herself and her family nutritious meals. Often, she would get a vague glazed expression on her face when I tried to gently make wellness suggestions. She was often miserable, depressed, and racked with guilt and just couldn't get out of the starting blocks to make basic health changes she knew would benefit herself and her family. In her mind putting her family first meant playing the martyr and placing herself on the back burner. Then she lost weight—too much weight—and without trying. She was actually happy until she got the diagnosis. She was sick and passed away in short order. Her family, especially her young daughter, was devastated. Shattered was more like it.

In the intervening years, I have cared for many thousands of people and have seen the same glazed expression often. It's the face of overwhelm, self-doubt, and a failure complex. In the many years since her passing I often think of Kim and her family and ask myself, "What if I could have cut through her guilt and really helped her?"

I am writing this book for the millions of men and women who may occasionally or permanently have that glazed look comprised of feelings of powerlessness and lack of hope in regard to their healthy weight, their fitness, their nutrition, and their mood and motivation.

This book will help readers understand the "missing link" of health and wellness which is that mindfulness and awareness of the present—rather than depression of the past or anxiety of the future—is the only arena where wellness can occur. The common affliction of "overwhelm" in our society is addressed within these pages and countered with a remarkably easy-breezy fitness and nutrition plan and activities to minimize or eliminate any guilt associated with proceeding down the path of change.

What else is in it for you? How about a doable, elegant, step-by-step plan for muscle gain and fat loss, an empowering guide to save huge swaths of time (and some cold hard cash) while reducing the one condition doctors of all stripes agree on as the leading cause of preventable disease today: inflammation. I endeavor to provide calming, nonjudgmental, one-second insights to positively and definitely move the meter of health in our world once and for all. I sincerely believe that if enough people digest and act on the myth-busting, common sense material in this book then, in the United States alone, we can save $1 trillion over ten years and reduce an untold number of travesties and tragedies as described in Kim's story. There are serious health problems in our Western society but the answers are surprisingly simple. I wrote this book for Kim, her family who loved her, and for men and women like her.

This book is not a diet book (I have never recommended a "diet" to anyone), a calorie counting book (I have never counted a calorie in my life or suggested anybody else count one), or a grunting, muscle-headed gym rat book (because my principles probably won't excite that population). This book is also not about having iron will power. It's not about that at all, rather my hope for you is to become addicted to the process of daily mini improvements for they are what truly constitute a happy, healthy life.

Remember the scene in the movie *What About Bob* where Richard Dreyfuss pompously recommends his book to a neurotic patient Bill Murray then hesitates as if he can't quite find the book he is looking for when his bookshelf has nothing but his book on it? That's me to you (minus the pomposity and the neurosis). I simply want you to win the head game of health. Wasn't it the cartoon character Pogo who said, "I have seen the enemy and it is us"? I want you to stop being your own worst enemy and see yourself the way you were truly designed to be: a superbly energetic, healthy super-star climber of life.

The Beta

The secret to wellness is climbing a mountain every day.

I have been a hiker and climber all my life. Sprinkled liberally in this book are mountain analogies and stories. Climbing and mountains make great metaphors. In mountaineering beta is jargon for climbing information given by someone who has already climbed the route. In the spirit of beta, I want to share something important. From one climber of life to another, the number one thing I want to get across to my readers, patients, and clients is never again to utter "I screwed up" or "I dropped the ball" or "I slipped" in regard to wellness. Self-flagellation is not helpful and in fact leads to guilt, overwhelm, and self-perpetuating poor habits. Be kind to yourself. Luxuriate yourself. (I love the verb luxuriate, it's one of those words that sounds like its definition.)

How about this: Just make a decision right now to improve or advance yourself a wee bit, either in head space, activity, or in nutrition. Just one of them. That's it. By doing one positive thing you shift your world. Perhaps unknowingly, one little positive change starts a domino effect in your internal and external world. A positive personal change stimulates your chemistry and quantum field fundamentally and starts inspired wellness momentum instantly. I'll show you how in the pages within. Inevitable stumbles will cause laughter rather than tears because the moment was seized. The truth becomes known: think long-term but act in the moment. Forget carpe diem because a day is too long. Seize the moment and use the Feet, Fork, and Fun principles to change your life. Consider me your Sherpa, guiding you along the dusty trail with your majestic snow-capped mountain (your health and fitness goals) squarely in view.

Every climber of life needs the best equipment. A common refrain in the hills is "there is no bad weather, only the wrong gear." What follows is some of the mental equipment and technology shared in this book.

Tone

Genetic Potential

3 × 3 × 3 = 6 Pack

The Dyno

Paleosity

Everest 70 Challenge

The Daily Dashboard

S.T.O.P. Method to Reboot

Fartlek

Empowered Mindfulness

C.R.A.P.

Preface

A One-Second Calling

Have you noticed that life can turn on a second? If you look back on your life to this point, I'll bet you can identify some moments that were truly momentous. Most probably some of these experiences you labeled good and some bad. I decided to be a doctor of chiropractic in one second. I knew my first marriage was over in one moment. I saw the curve of the earth from the summit of Mount Everest in one second. I cut my son's umbilical cord with a pair of scissors in one second. What about you? If you agree that moments make up our entire existence, then you may accept the significance of a reboot or reset when it comes to Feet, Fork, and Fun wellness principles. The following story illustrates the preparatory lead up to the moment I decided to become a doctor. My point is to share the idea that with every momentous turning point event there is a sizable lead up. The importance lies in the realization that achieving your goal of healthy living and fitness may have been rattling around in your subconscious for years. Act before it's too late. It was too late for Kim.

I was heavily into running in my early years. School was only a concern because it provided a platform for me to run track and cross-country. I brought a stack of school books home just to placate my parents. I just wanted to run.

I was twelve years old when I watched the 1972 Summer Olympics and screamed as Frank Shorter won the marathon gold for the United States. I was definitely fired up. I was inspired by the physical endurance and I was inspired by the mental tenacity to run twenty-six miles at a sub-five-minutes-per-mile pace. I was inspired to learn what it took to achieve one's human potential.

Unmotivated by traditional school requirements, I devoured the subjects of nutrition, physiology, psychology, and endurance training in periodicals, such as *Runner's World* magazine and every book or journal I could grab at nearby University of Rhode Island library.

It occurred to me as a fifteen-year-old freshman that a career in health care was in my future—physical therapy kind of made sense, as I could see myself working with and helping other athletes.

Flash forward four years. As a college sophomore I had just finished cross-country season when I couldn't run another step. My body had become a mess of dysfunctional pain, numbness, tingling, and weakness. I had run my second marathon at age eighteen in under three hours—a very decent time and a lifetime goal for good runners at any age, but my body had collapsed soon afterward. Too much training at a young age, I surmised.

Nine months went by and still I couldn't run a step. I saw "the best sports medicine doctor" in the county. Each visit, the ritual ended with a shot of cortisone. There was no change and no benefit. When he started to talk about exploratory surgery, I never went back. This was before arthroscopic surgery, and the scar that I had seen on several other athletes was about eight inches long and these people seemed worse to me (and old).

What I decided to do was go to a chiropractor. I was referred by buddies in the running community and although I had never heard the word "chiropractic" or "chiropractor" and was clueless about what they did, I made an appointment for the simple reason that he was also a runner.

Later that very same day, I went out and ran... and ran... and ran. I could not believe it. I could run again. I ran five miles that day when I had not been able to run a step in nine months. I had some minor twinges but no pain—a miracle for me.

I went back to Dr. Recor the next week. I had one hand on the doorknob and was about to turn it... when, here it comes—a huge mountainous moment in my life: A thought flash. I could be a chiropractor. I should be a chiropractor. Hey, I will become a chiropractor and help people just like me.

I finished up my BA degree at Rhode Island College, received my Doctor of Chiropractic Degree from Palmer College of Chiropractic in 1986, and started practicing in Warwick, Rhode Island, in August 1987.

I participated in over a quarter-million patient interactions then sold my practice to concentrate on reaching a larger audience through speaking, writing, and coaching. My purpose was to help as many people as possible reach their full health potential.

My professional calling became manifest because of one second of insight followed by action.

Looking back on life's adventures has taught me that paying attention to moments—or seconds if you want to quantify the moment—makes all the difference in our human experience.

I will wager you have some of your own magic moments.

My great hope for you is to fall in love with the moment, the present. The past is history and the future a dream so all we really have is the now. Fall in love with it. Develop a love relationship with the present because that is the only place we exist. By having an intimate relationship with the present we can cut through societal and internally created BS and finally experience our healthy weight, great energy, deep restful rejuvenating sleep, optimal physical fitness, and prevention and stabilization of disease... and have a blast in the process.

Caution: Mountain Analogy.

In my first attempt to climb Mount Everest in 2007 there was a dude on the team who was pretty carefree. He made plenty of mistakes but none fatal, thankfully. He joked around a lot and had fun. I, on the other hand, was never comfortable. I was wound up and negatively stressed. I was terrified of the climb to come. My friend, we'll call him Nick, rebooted from his mistakes, made the summit, and had fun in the process. I did not reboot, did not have fun, and for many different reasons did not summit that year. I've never forgotten the lesson. In fact, I used the lesson for the next year of training and planning and successfully summited the top of the world the very next year.

Part One

Tone: Get It, Keep It

1910: Life is the expression of tone. Tone is expressed in functions by the normal elasticity, activity, strength and excitability of the various organs as observed in a state of health.—D.D. Palmer

2016: Tone is our natural human state. Tone is the optimal balance of physical, chemical, and emotional lifestyle choices modulated by our inborn genetic potential.—The Author

One-Second Wellness

You're a ghost driving a meat-coated skeleton made from stardust riding a rock hurtling through space. Fear nothing.—Unknown

A Day in the Life

5:45 A.M.

Catherine's alarm blared. She felt leaden like she had just fallen asleep even though, by her reckoning, she had six hours under her belt, about average she realized.

6:15 A.M.

"I've got to get moving," she mumbled to herself as she tugged and pulled the zipper of her beige pencil skirt. Like all her fave outfits this one had become uncomfortably tight. "That's it. I am definitely going on a diet and restarting my exercise this week."

7:15 A.M.

Zoning out to a news talk show where people were yelling, stopping briefly to go to commercial before ratcheting up the belligerence again, Catherine realized with a start that she hadn't eaten anything again. Almost on cue, she pulled into the drive-through lane at the local donut and coffee joint and, remembering her earlier desire to start dieting and exercising, she scanned the menu deciding on an egg white and cheddar microwaved sandwich, a one percent milk, and another regular coffee.

7:45 A.M.

The first two rows of the parking lot at work were full so she drove around twice before deciding to squeeze her car into a too small space in the front row, saving her nine seconds of walking to the front door.

12:22 P.M.

Thursdays were lunch-n-learn days at the high tech firm where Catherine worked. The meeting room was in a building about a quarter mile away and, afraid of being the last one there, she took the shuttle even though she felt a bit embarrassed she wasn't walking. She prepared a salad of mixed greens, cherry tomatoes, and a green pepper slice then ladled on some creamy Italian and made a sandwich of ham, provolone, mustard, and wheat bread. She washed it down with a perfectly chilled diet cola. She shuttled back to her building with coworker Joan because she didn't want to interrupt their strategizing session even as they boarded the elevator to the third floor together.

5:45 P.M.

She grabbed some hummus, pita chips, a glass of pinot, and headed for the living room to ritually watch the news from six to seven o'clock. At seven, Catherine reluctantly turned the TV off before the trashy Hollywood gossip shows began and started dinner of frozen peas and hamburgers, milk for the kids, and water and another pinot for mom and dad. The TV was back on for the 'Sox game after dinner and the kids filed into their rooms to putz on their devices while mom and dad did dishes, tidied up the house, chatted, and passed out after the 11:30 news.

The next day was essentially identical for Catherine and her family, as was the day after that.

Let's recap. We arise and operate our vehicle to work where we sit and operate electronic devices in an artificial space with other space aliens. Then we go home to muddle through with slightly more familiar space aliens till we get the chance to not sleep enough, then barely get up to do it all over again. To fuel this, we eat who-knows-what from who-knows-where as long as we can get it "now." Houston, we have a problem.

Health is a shedding process.—The Author

One-Second Universal Truths

Forget about feeling like you have to know it all. You, Catherine, and the world do not need more facts, figures, and random pop opinions from "experts," many of whom have an agenda to sell you stuff. Leave that idea. The world needs to embrace Universal Truths. Universal Truths are simple enough for both elite and outcast to understand and manifest. The Universal Truths shared in this book include (1) health comes from within; (2) optimal health is available to everyone who takes personal responsibility for it; (3) we only have control of the present; (4) little things are big things when they are habits; (5) health exists in three dimensions of Feet, Fork, and Fun; (6) an attention to and a balance of these dimensions is vital for optimal health; (7) how we live our lives can interfere with the natural state of tone; and (8) achieving and maintaining tone is mainly a shedding process rather than an accumulation process.

People are healing machines once they get themselves out of the way.
—The Author

Warning: Mind Blower Alert

I know what you may be thinking: One-Second Wellness? Sounds like a gimmick to me! You can't possibly get healthy in one second, or even a month.

If you are of the doubting variety I can sympathize, but try this on for size: We have about seventy trillion cells in the human body (70,000,000,000,000). If you don't believe this fact start counting now and in a few lifetimes you will see that science is indeed correct. Get this: every SECOND each cell (of the 70 million) is performing six million vital functions (6,000,000). That's not all by a long shot. This is the one that blows my mind. Every cell knows what ALL the other cells are doing. They communicate. That's why a big toe cell is not trying to be a red blood cell or a liver cell is not attempting function on the lung team. Adding to this amazingly complex orchestrated symphony is the fact that cells are continually dying, being removed and recycled, and new cells created in their place, with most of the body being replaced in a few months or less. Self-healing, self-regulating, self-maintaining, and conscious all in a second. I humbly suggest the reader keep an open mind that maybe a moment in time is more than we mortals suspect.

15

It's the brain and nervous system that runs the above miracle show, but unfortunately it can be interfered with. It can screw up and not work like Mother Nature intended. The interference is in three types, or dimensions: physical, chemical, and emotional. Some aspects of these dimensions we humans have control of and some we don't. My purpose in this timeless contribution to the world's body of knowledge that you are holding is to (1) identify interferences to health that people have control over each day, minute, and second and (2) suggest easy, step-by-step, elegant ways to minimize interferences in order to work in harmony with innate bodily function. The result is the highest version of the healthiest YOU expressing its innate fabulousness.

Your Daily Dashboard

I like trucks. The older, classier, and more worn, the better. My favorite vehicle I ever owned was an ancient, cranky Land Rover Defender with no creature comforts at all. It sported the swagger to drive through or over anything in its path in mud, snow, or sand with its four-wheel drive, monstrous tires, and high clearance.

I drove it for many years, then my son Kurt drove it for years, then I drove it again for more years. The spartan dashboard on the beast revealed only the essentials: speedometer, tachometer, gas level, odometer, voltage, oil.

A momentary glance down gave the operator all the information needed while descending a steep sand hill or traversing a mud pit of unknown depth. A glance at a dashboard gives one-second feedback so you can make decisions.

Alert: Mountain Analogy

My dashboard in May 2008 was the only thing between life and a cold, lonely death high on the Southeast Ridge of Mount Everest. My dashboard was a virtual one, and every climbing second I scanned and re-scanned for insight and solutions to questions of survival at 29,000 feet—the same elevation as a cruising 747. Several frozen corpses of previous expedition members reminded my altitude-addled mind of the severity of poor choices.

Are all my crampons in the ice?

Is my safety loop and Jumar engaged on the fixed rope?

Do I need an energy gel?

Is it safe to stop and drink?

Do I need to vent my 'pits, pants, or jacket to prevent frostbite, or do I need to button up to protect against losing fingers, toes, or some other vital appendage?

The most important questions and answers were in the mental realm as high altitude famously disrupts decision making and judgment:

Am I stumbling, suggesting high altitude cerebral edema?

If I speak out loud, are my words garbled?

Is my breathing labored (normal at high altitude even without red-lined exertion) or am I frothing blood with each breath, suggesting high-altitude pulmonary edema?

Am I concentrating adequately or am I am a laissez-faire dead man walking (another symptom of HACE)?

Am I with it, or am I losing it?

My mental dashboard on the mountain was my instantaneous connection to life while inhabiting an inhospitable deadly place. It forced me to live in the one place we all exist: The moment, the present.

We all need an awareness dashboard, even at sea level on a seventy-five-degree sunny day while driving to work. The upshot of checking in regularly with your wellness dashboard goes well beyond the physical, chemical, and emotional health and leads directly to "fun, fun, fun." It simply feels good to luxuriate yourself, especially if you are replacing poor habits with good ones, a classic win-win.

I remind patients, audience members, and coaching clients that little things are big things in disguise, and little things are really big things when they are habits. Checking in often with your daily dashboard ensures implementation and maintenance of great healthy habits.

One-Second Wellness is all about having a love relationship with the present moment.

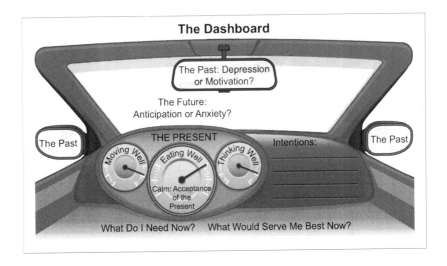

C.R.A.P.

As a doctor participating in over a quarter-million healing encounters with all kinds of people from CEOs of major companies to homeless people and from kids just hours old to energetic oldsters of 102, I believe that the reason people do not participate in even simple, positive health behaviors is a combination of four things, C.R.A.P.:

- Complacency—bored (and lazy).
- Rationalization—"I would do it but my favorite *Seinfeld* re-run is on."
- Apathy—"I don't have any control so I am not going to do anything."
- Procrastination—"I will start next week."

My mother corrected me endlessly whenever I used the word "crap," and for good reason. It grates, could be defined as in poor taste, and is a low level swear word. The only reason I use it is because it serves as a harsh reminder of the worthlessness of the behaviors spelled out in the acronym. The four attributes of C.R.A.P. are the reasons many people do not succeed in what they know will be healthy for themselves and their families. The four C.R.A.P. attributes serve as a default position for too many of us too often, and all are related to not living in the present. Some succumb more than others, but all of us human knuckleheads at one time or another fall prey to the insidious waste of C.R.A.P.. Watch out.

C.R.A.P. not only is bad news for wellness and health but also results in lowered self-esteem and neophobia, or fear of making a change. It gets harder and harder to break out and make positive health changes the longer people are in the rut of C.R.A.P.. By the way, a rut is a coffin with the ends bashed out.

Having any fear is no fun, but neophobia is particularly debilitating, becoming a vicious circle of lowered human potential, and in regard to health, the fear of making necessary changes can manifest as crisis across every stratum of life—physical, mental, financial, social—everything.

Health Guilt Is Killing Us

I don't know if you have ever smoked cigarettes. I did. I smoked four of them in a row once while sitting in a humongous beech tree near my bus stop when I was eleven. Those four cigs sucked literally and figuratively, but that's beside the point. Trying to get people to stop smoking or stop any other unhealthy activity has an interesting history. For many years it was thought if we can scare people enough they will stop. It certainly seemed logical but guess what? Scare care has never worked. With cigarette smokers, how many times have they seen diseased lungs on a cigarette pack? Or have heard disease statistics associated with smoking? It does not end smoking. Smokers feel bad then pick up another cig to feel better. It seems insane to nonsmokers but it remains a predictable pattern unless the pain of the habit becomes overwhelming and people adopt a new healthier habit or get help to change the reality. Similarly, guilt-ridden alcoholics sometimes drink again because they feel bad about drinking. Heroin addicts can relapse.

Quite probably the most common example of the "guilt, fail, guilt, fail again" cycle relates to food. Many people observed in my practice had a relationship with food that was firmly in the addiction camp. The issue was sometimes overeating itself or attachment to a particular substance—more often than not sugar. The same cycle as the alcoholic was evident: eat sugar, feel bad about it, because you feel bad, you eat more sugar. Most people know the right thing to do and have heard all the scare-care recommendations, but they feel better when they use food as a medicine—at least for a short time.

As a former purveyor of health guilt as a young doctor, I saw the light and observed that people will follow a plan if it appears reasonable, truthful, and doable... and patients will have fun doing it. Negative scare care labeling is the opposite of fun. The antidote for health guilt is focus on the present, on the "now," and doing one positive thing or eliminate one negative at a time. One-second living.

"What would serve me best right now?"—You

"What do I need now?"—You

Hoka Hey!

Do you burn the midnight oil in deep thought about the meaning of life and the philosophic debate of impermanence and reality? Crazy Horse apparently did. Crazy Horse, who lived from 1842 to 1877, was a warrior, military leader, a folk hero, chief of the Oglala Sioux, backed up Neil Young, and was a big reason why General Custer had a bad day at Little Big Horn. His famous quote "Hoka Hey" roughly translates to "It is a good day to die."

Caution: Mountain story to hopefully illustrate the point ahead.

I first heard "Hoka Hey" when I was scared witless while standing on a flat area of stone the size of a teeny bedroom at 11,000 feet on the Grand Teton in the Wyoming Rocky Mountains, making a climbing attempt with friends Bob and Scott in 2001. Scott uttered the phrase. Bob and I both hated it.

We were at a pitch on the classic Owen-Spalding route where we would be hanging on a flake of granite by our fingertips with 3,000 feet of air below us while shuffling crablike on the vertical rock to the relative safety of the next belay.

I will not forget the moment nor the phrase anytime soon. I have returned to it time and again over the years and have found it to be both powerful and calming. We are all going to leave our bodies at some point and cannot choose the time and the place, so why would I not live my best life right now? Why not live to my highest health potential now? Why not go for it? Why not share my gifts with the world to the best of my ability? Why not begin now where you stand (preferably not on a slab of stone high in the air or charging into battle on a war pony with

Springfield and tomahawk in tow)? Why not live your dream now? Why not be the healthiest you can be now? Instead of, "What's in your wallet?" I think we should be asking, "What's on my dashboard?" "What would serve me best right now?" "What do I need now?" and then exclaiming "Hoka Hey! You big beautiful world."

Drugs-R-Us

It is well established that in order to be successful at pretty much anything, you have to take complete responsibility for your life. Jack Canfield, coauthor of *The Chicken Soup* series of books and success philosopher extraordinaire, in his opus *The Success Principles*, says taking 100% responsibility is the most important facet of a successful life. In fact, he puts it on the first page of the book.

Nowhere is demanding and taking full responsibility more important than in the arena of personal wellness and, more particularly, the use and misuse of medication.

Right across the street from my chiropractic office was a dialysis center, and I cared for some of the nurses and management there. The dialysis nurses had to hook patients with kidney failure to the machines daily to do the job that the kidneys normally do, cleanse and filter the blood. The workers continuously told me that the vast majority of dialysis patients ruined their kidneys from the use of over-the-counter NSAIDs, or non-steroidal anti-inflammatory drugs, like Advil, Motrin, and the ilk. Taking any over-the-counter, under-the-counter, or contacting and handling any chemical substance for that matter is not advisable unless the person has done due diligence and researched the use and misuse of said chemical. To be healthy as citizens we need to be aware objectively and without emotion of the risk vs. reward of ingestion or contact of any chemical, medication, or unknown substance. Another sad note on NSAIDs is that about 16,000 Americans die each year from taking them. Over-the-counter doesn't mean safe at all.

Many of us have heard about today's massive increase in heroin addicts and overdoses—much of which is related to doctors and dentists who over-prescribe narcotic pain killers. Later, when prescriptions dry up, many of the addicted turn to the much cheaper, more available, and deadly heroin—with or without fentanyl. The sad demise of musicians from Elvis to Prince illustrate the problem. Sadly, the latter was reported to be drug and alcohol free for most of his life. I have lost a niece to this scourge. Even if people have not switched to heroin, there has been an increase of 700% in the death rate in my personal age group of 55 to 64 from prescribed pain killer overdoses. Again, before taking any chemical or medication, learn about it and take responsibility for it. Own it, good or bad. Even when your doctor says you absolutely need a certain drug, research, research, research. Your doctors are your coaches and advisors but you are president and CEO of you.

Antidepressants, though necessary in many cases, increase the childhood suicide rate, a fact that has been buried for years by pharmaceutical companies who garner huge profits. Hospital-acquired infections kill twelve people an hour. It goes on and on.

Taking responsibility, minimizing contact, and living a wellness lifestyle is the only cure for shenanigans involving Big Pharma. I don't think there is any other way because there is just too much money involved. I am not saying you will never have to take a prescribed drug in your life just that it should be as a result of thoughtful research and rational decision making.

YOU, YOU, YOU, YOU!—chant at basketball games after opposing player commits a foul.

What's that? You say you're not a doctor? That's great news because it's not any doctor's job to keep you well. It's yours. In generations past, you listened to the doctor and you followed what he said like it was gospel. That was then.

Use your doctors as trusted guides, but be the king or queen of you. Accept and relish that responsibility. Is it God's job to keep you well? Nope, it's You, You, You. Is your health and wellness determined by your genetics, either good or bad? No way again, our genetics play a role with health, but it's how we live our life that determines how our genetics are expressed. The fascinating study of epigenetics supports this. It turns out that health is mostly related to our environment and HOW we live our life in that environment. In the insect world, a worker bee and queen bee are genetically identical with the same DNA but the queen becomes a queen by being bathed in a unique stew of bee goop. As humans, how we live our lives has been hypothesized to be passed on for multiple generations. In other words: live a wellness lifestyle today and your future grandbabies are better off.

Poor health usually has no symptoms, at least at the beginning. It's painless... for a while. As a matter of fact, the first symptom in thirty percent of first heart attacks is death. Painless... then you croak. Healthy doesn't mean you never get sick. In actuality, after a viral or bacterial illness, for example, you are actually healthier afterward because the properly functioning genius of the body produces antibodies that recognize the invading organism and attack and kill it the next time it shows up in your internal environment. If you spend the night in the bathroom after eating some bad oysters does it mean you're sick? Actually, no. The healthy body eliminates the poison while the unhealthy can't... and gets sicker. Before speaking in Iowa a while back I apparently let my resistance down because I developed a fever. Thankfully I got through my presentation without passing out but I was thankful because my healthy body was elevating the temperature to "burn out" the invading organism. It was also an opportunity to reflect and learn more fully what steps I can take to stay well. Some folks have been indoctrinated to take a dangerous drug, acetaminophen (i.e., Tylenol), to artificially reduce a fever—inadvertently short circuiting their own genetic potential. Do your research in this regard.

The good news is that human beings are healing machines. We all have a secret weapon in the health game and it's not some lotion, potion, or pill. It's been freely working its magic since before you were born. This miraculously incredible magical inborn healing ability is called genetic intelligence or genetic potential—others call it God within. Genetic potential self-heals and self-regulates. Genetic potential is the power that made the body—turning two cells into 70 trillion. Genetic potential works like a charm but can be interfered with.

Mountain Moments

How do you climb Mount Everest or lose fifty pounds? One step at a time.

How do you get maximally well and healthy? One moment at a time.

I love all things mountain. I love the challenge and exhilaration of climbing them, even if I have to turn around for one reason or another and climb it another day. I love mountains framed on my walls, pinned on my Pinterest, stacked in my book shelves, and vocalized on my playlists. I surmise they are popular with me and others because they illustrate a metaphor for big, hairy, audacious undertakings as well as overcoming nearly overwhelming obstacles.

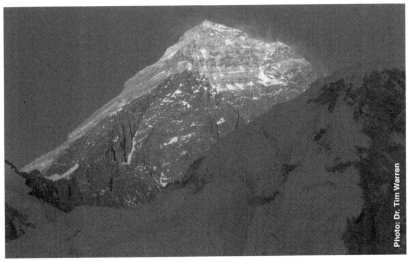

Mount Everest, 2007

As you traverse the pages in this book and plunge your ice axe into the content and ascend the mountain of health and wellness, pay attention to the feelings of well-being and self-satisfaction that come as a result of making great health-promoting decisions in the moment. These are the metaphorical steps of climbing your own Everest of health.

The idea of one step at a time or one foot in front of the other makes it easy to visualize and experience success in any endeavor. Each step climbed is a mountain moment. Each second spent making good health decisions and discarding old poor health habits allows you to spend time on the summit of health. We will win some and lose some. No problemo on this one. Remember, this book is for losers... who are winners simultaneously. The big picture is shortening the reboot time.

Make Yourself Hard to Kill

The purpose of training is to make yourself hard to kill.—The Author

Will you be a decrepit and feeble old goat or will you be an aged, wise, respected, and vital family hero? Will you be the Gandalf the Grey of your 'hood? Or perhaps the Jedi Knight of the family reunion is more your thing? I am all about training you for either, just know that it involves an open clear mind, a willingness to learn, and the chutzpa to stick to it. This is about training for your personal and family wellness. Making health habits easy, breezy, and doable isn't magic but it is training. It's about training for your 120th birthday.

Super Important Info Ahead. This section has the most important information you, young Padawan learner, need to "get." If you only read this small section you will have gotten your money's worth from this book. Internalize this part, act on it, and you will immediately have a long beard, a cool staff, and a stylish wizard's hat.

Wellness and optimum health and fitness exist in a balance of understanding and implementing the three dimensions of Feet, Fork, and Fun. Each of these dimensions makes up an equally important third of the mountain.

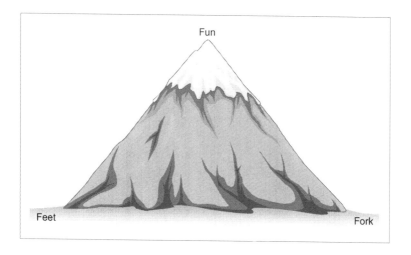

The FEET dimension is How You Use Your Body. It encompasses sleep; cardiovascular health; strength; flexibility in muscles, tendons, and ligaments; and posture.

The FORK dimension is defined as What We Do or Do Not Put Into Our Body. This vital area encompasses nutrition but also involves the quality of air and water and other environmental factors with which we may come in contact.

The last of the three dimensions of life is the psychological or emotional or FUN dimension. The FUN dimension involves the mind–body connection. The Fun dimension of health is stimulated and enhanced by... get this... learning stuff! Right this moment you are enhancing your Fun dimension, and your health, simply by reading this book. So cool! In my lectures and presentations around the country this dimension is my favorite by far. For some, this dimension may be the hardest to understand but in my experience it is the most important to harness for healthy living. Once you peruse and absorb through Chapter Eight I am confident you will be an expert in FUN. It's so important I put FUN at the summit.

Summary:

Feet: How we use our body.

Fork: What we do and do not put into our body.

Fun: The mind–body connection.

There are healthy positive items to maximize daily in these three dimensions, additionally there are negative unhealthy items to minimize each day. We get healthier by accentuating the positive good stuff and minimizing the negative bad stuff. It's as simple as that. Moments of truth or moments of choice are those times when you can go either way. I think you should go the right way because then you can brag about your results, tell the world about this book, and I can get a Medal of Freedom in 2026 because I saved the country $1 trillion health care dollars.

Your Daily Summit

Mountain Story With Meaningful Message: When someone asks me about climbing Mt. Everest either in one of my slideshows or while standing next to me in a bathroom, they are usually referring to what it was like on the summit. Besides the intense fear, penetrating cold, misery of a seventy-day expedition, uncertainty of surviving the descent, and the wasting of the body and mind at high altitude, the summit is a pretty fantabulous experience. Summit week on Everest in late May is like the Super Bowl of climbing albeit steeped in physical and mental uncertainty, pain, and fear. You spend two months above 17,000 feet in dangerous remote camps preparing body, mind, and equipment simply to put your team in a position to attempt the summit of the biggest mountain on the planet. The weather and conditions have to be just right to follow through. All your focus and energy is on the basics of survival. It's a competition but not among climbers. It's competition with yourself, nature, and your decision making. You have the weather window and the strength for just one shot at it. A million things can go wrong and yet when you are fortunate enough to get to the top of your mountain and gaze out at magnificent views—there is nothing like the feeling of accomplishment. You realize on some level that you are a changed person for life. It is the feeling of being one with nature and creation. The Everest climber becomes deeply humble and emotional after enduring and surviving the test.

I experience similar warm and fuzzy feelings (minus the tears) when I make good health decisions day by day and decision by decision and especially the morning. A first thing in the morning wellness ritual sets the tone for the day. It gets me supremely juiced for my work day and for accomplishment in my life. How would you feel starting your day with a personal summit? I highly recommend a first thing in the morning daily summit for supplying ample jet fuel to the rest of your day.

How cool would it be to summit a really tall, majestic, stunningly beautiful mountain each morning and throughout the day? Imagine having fun first thing in the morning just by making healthy choices. For some folks, the default is to meet the day with a groan, and the day doesn't get much better from there. There is no inspirational juice in that scenario.

Maybe you know people who get up late on work days and mope into the bathroom, then mope into the kitchen for coffee, then plop in front of the news where for every thirty minutes of bad news that is injected into your brain, there are also fifteen minutes of mind-numbing commercials that are stared at in a fog of nonaction. Next comes a mad rush to get dressed and the kids fed and out the door—and darn, forgot to eat anything. A quick stop for a greasy pseudo-breakfast sandwich and on to work where you can guess how the day progresses.

Instead I propose a summit day every morning. It might look something like this, and it will not take any extra time from your already packed life. Try this morning on for size.

Make the bed (yes, make the damn bed!) with a 3 × 5 card on the pillow (more on this in a moment) and have five big swallows of water and coffee or tea black. Your favorite educational, objective, non-anger-inducing smart person news radio show is on the speaker, such as NPR, or an inspirational or educational audiobook. As soon as you have looked out the window and noticed how peaceful and beautiful it is outside and meditated a moment on the miracle of green things growing, you step on a wobble board or a BOSU ball for some brain–body movement stimulation which gets both fired up, followed by three sets of perfect-form Super Brain Yoga maneuvers (you will learn the particulars later down the road or go to www.drtimwarren.com and check out the video section).

Now that you are inspired, motivated, and warmed up how about a "finisher"? Three fifteen- to sixty-second planks (descriptions in Chapter Six, Feet) and zap your abs and core, and a walkabout (a Dr. Tim Walkabout is a five- to thirty-minute stroll outside at your choice of variable speeds and must include The Bad Wedding Dance Four-Step and a few deep cleansing breaths), if time permits, before a body- and mind-enhancing breakfast choice—for example, a protein shake with a non-sugared fruit juice base, a handful of spinach, and a banana thrown in. By the way, a muscle shake like this takes longer to drink than to make and can be easily taken to work in a shaker cup.

Your spouse or spouse equivalent and the kids or kid equivalent are well fed in similar fashion, everybody is on time, and your chemistry, confidence, energy, and attitude are rocking. Dunkin' Donuts might not be happy, but all 70 trillion cells in your body are very, very happy with you, and most importantly, you are feeling good about you.

Chapter One: Brain Train Exercise

Write your ideal morning routine beginning with making your bed, include the Feet, Fork, and Fun dimensions.

How a 3 × 5 Card Will Change Your Life

By the way, why a 3 × 5 card? It's your goal card! But it's more than a goal card because it's your INTENTION CARD. The ubiquitous 3 × 5 is easy to carry and refer to all day (mine is neon pink and inhabits my iPhone case so it peeks at me all day). You simply write your intentions for the next seventy days (the time it takes for a Mt. Everest expedition). It's simple to discard and make a new one if the goals cease to resonate or get stale while limiting the goal focusing to what you can write on one side. Any more than that is a mind muddle and not useful.

What if you looked at your intentions every morning, lunch time, and night? What if you did this every day? What if you only did half of it? Would that be easy, doable? Very much so, as long as complacency, rationalization, apathy, and procrastination—and/or neophobia—are not allowed to slide under the crack of your door that always exists. C.R.A.P. should not be allowed to rear its success-sapping, venomous head and the intention card is a weapon of choice.

At the end of the day read your card one last time and place it on your nightstand or a place where it will not be missed because the next morning, first thing upon arising, you will make your bed and read the card again. I have found that if I fail to make my bed first thing in the morning the rest of my day has a tendency to look like my rumpled sheets with pillows all askew. I do not want any chance of rumpled or askew thinking to infect my consciousness or subconsciousness. Practice congruency.

Stuff goes wrong sometimes, right? Stuff will go wrong every day. We fail every day. This is normal. I have news for you. Blowing it and failing is not a problem, and as a matter of fact, it should be relished as it is all part of life's good stuff. It is an opportunity to grow and learn. You will be late for work some days without having a healthy breakfast. So what? Learn from it and move right on. It's what you do most of the time that counts. Here's the secret: by having summits every morning, the successes mount throughout the day and the failures minimize and, even when you do inevitably flub, you forgive yourself and laugh. Summit wisdom in action.

In my hiking, climbing, and fitness life of over five decades, I seem to remember the bad weather trips, the wrong gear trips, or the bad teammate trips better than the ones where everything went perfectly. I realize now it's because people grow in adversity as long as it's not overwhelming (such as a PTSD situation). I adapted, grew, learned, became more Gandalf-like, and then usually ended up with a rash of way more compelling stories to tell.

It is said that human motivation is steeped in avoiding pain and seeking pleasure. I propose embracing pain (for learning purposes) then enjoying the hell out of the pleasure.—The Author

---

Chapter One: Points to Ponder

1. Your body consists of 70 trillion cells each performing 6 million functions per second while simultaneously communicating with all the others. Do you think you should pour soda on it?

2. Moments are precious.

3. Use your wellness dashboard for instant guidance in the drive of life.

4. C.R.A.P. and neophobia stink. Stay aware.

5. Hoka Hey! If it is in fact a good day to die, then why not kick some butt now? If not now, when?

6. It's all your responsibility. Embrace this as it's good news.

7. Take one small tenacious step at a time in your chosen direction. After all, it's your intention.

CHAPTER TWO

Tone: The Mount Everest of Health

Natural forces within us are the true healers of disease.—Hippocrates

Tone: The Mount Everest of Health

Have you ever seen those TV advertisements for credit scores that have a gauge to instantly see what your number is? It implies that if you make a purchase, payment, or some financial decision then the number will go up or down accordingly. Health decisions and habits are the same way. Nobody became obese overnight just like an Olympic athlete didn't get in shape in a day. Health decisions good and bad are on a cumulative basis of moment by moment and day to day accounting. What is the goal of wellness? I'm here to tell you the intention of health is tone. I am not talking about toned muscles although buffness inside and out can be a component of your tone. Tone is a state of overall physical, chemical, and emotional balance. Tone is you paying attention to Feet, Fork, and Fun not just in the moment but for a lifetime.

Homeostasis is defined as the constant inborn balancing of functional processes in response to the body's environment in order to maintain health. Your genetic intelligence at work. Homeostasis and tone are cousins.

A simple example of homeostasis would be if you are inside your house on a brisk winter day and do not put a jacket on and you step outside, your body goes through myriad changes—shivering, goose bumps, circulation changes to the skin—in response to the stress of colder weather. Your body does what it has to to maintain balance and life.

Likewise, when you go inside your toasty home, your body automatically adjusts again internally—changes the circulation, changes the function of the body to get back to that normal base temperature.

Mind Blower Alert. In my almost forty years in the health biz, the more I study and learn about the body, the more it stuns and amazes me that people are alive in the first place. Wowser. This may be why I can't stop guilting my elderly pop for his deep love of cream-filled donuts.

Your Highest Health Potential

Tone is achieved by allowing your inborn genetic intelligence to do its magic while heightening or enhancing its miraculous function by Moving Right, Eating Right, and Thinking Right. This is your to do list for Feet, Fork, and Fun. Tone is our three-dimensional human responsibility to honor the perfection within by treating our body vessel in the healthiest way possible. Tone is a heightened healthy state and it can be fleeting if it's not viewed as a continuous, never ending process. Tone is a higher state of physical, chemical, and emotional existence. Another way to describe it is your highest health potential. Tone is a most worthy intention. The three dimensions of body, chemistry, and mind—Chapter Five, Feet: Why; Chapter Six, Feet: How; Chapter Seven, Fork; and Chapter Eight, Fun—are integral to the development and goal of tone.

Wellness and tone are always in flux. We are always under construction. Tone and homeostasis never end as long as life exists. It's not supposed to end. All of us are on a wellness continuum. Visualize a vertical multi-rung ladder reaching to the top of the Mount Everest of health. Healthy lifestyle choices are rewarded with another rung climbed with everything we do either enhancing or deteriorating tone and health. Our tone is a function of a constantly shifting ebb and flow of innate bodily function (homeostatic fluctuations) of inborn power with one relentless purpose: maintaining your genetic potential. How you choose to live your life in a perfect world accentuates and honors your inborn healing power.

Tucked away in our subconscious is an idyllic dream. We see ourselves on a long expedition to the most beautiful mountain in the world. We are walking through vibrant hills and valleys with beautiful pastoral scenes playing out all around us. We drink in the scenes of everyday life. We see children playing, the green and brown fields tilled and harvested, rushing streams, smoke wafting above a stone chimney, and the scents on the wind are of forest and ritual incense.

But uppermost in our minds is the final destination. The mountain summit. On a particular day at a particular time we will pull ourselves up to the very top. Bands will play and prayer flags will wave and it will be glorious. When we get there our life will be complete and have meaning. Once we get there all our dreams will come true. We become restless on the trail. We can't wait to get to the top. The minutes and days and years drag.

"When we get the summit that will be it!" we exclaim. "When I'm 21." "When I get the 560SL Mercedes." "When my son graduates from college." "When the mortgage gets paid off." "When I retire I will be happy for the rest of my life."

Sooner or later we have to realize there is no mountain summit, no one place to finally arrive at. The joy and our life's purpose is the journey. The summit is a dream.

"Enjoy the climb" is a good admonition. It isn't the burdens of climbing that drive people mad it is guilt over the past and fear of the future. Both rob us of today.

Therefore, stop whining about the blister on your heel and counting the hours. Instead, hike more trails, see more mountains, watch more sunsets, go barefoot more, laugh more, and covet less. Life must be lived fully as we traverse the trail. The summit will come soon enough.

Q: "Hey Dr. Tim, when I get tone can I binge watch TV for the rest of my life?"

A: "Can you brush, floss, and oil pull your mouth squeaky clean once and then never have to brush again?"

It's impossible to eat well, move well, and think well for a couple of days and become magically toned forever. Nope, tone's a lifestyle. Good habits for body and mind have to be done and redone for the rest of your life, or at least as long as you want to rock-n-roll.

Tone is done daily, not to be confused with actress Tyne Daly.

Tone. Nature's health insurance. —The Author

The Triune of Life

Our physiology, or bodily function, is designed to run at 100% efficiency 24/7. Bodily functions don't stop, ever, because that would be the next adventure otherwise known as death. While sleeping, our body repairs and recharges the system. This self-healing, self-regulating system is also part of your genetic intelligence. You don't even have to think about it, it just works, but in order to have 100% life in the body, you have to have three things:

- 100% matter—you have to have all the parts, like a liver, spleen, eyeball, and those cute little piggies of yours. (Phantom pain is an interesting phenomenon in which, for years after a person loses a limb, they can experience pain in a part that no longer remains. This is the genetic intelligence trying to communicate to a part that is not even there.)

- 100% energy.

- 100% communication.

This triune of innate function is modulated by our nervous system, made up of the brain, the spinal cord, and the nerves. It makes us perfect. We are perfect inside when genetic intelligence controls a person with 100% of matter, energy, and communication. It's important to realize that you can have interference to the perfect nature of innate intelligence especially in the communication aspect. In chiropractic we call the interference subluxation.

When there is overwhelming negative stress in the Feet or Fork or Fun areas, or commonly all three, the body does not function and communicate like Mother Nature intended it to. Sooner or later health deteriorates. The result can be pain, disease, illness, dysfunction, or susceptibility to infection, but the bottom line is we are not at 100% potential for health. Quite commonly, no symptoms or pain initially occur, which means people are unaware they have diminished health potential. Our innate does its best with what it has to work with but the system is off-kilter. This dude is losing it in the tone department.

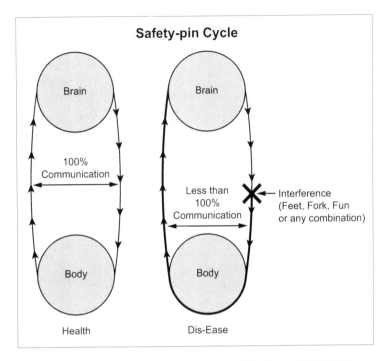

At this point of bodily dysfunction, I would channel Jeff Bridges in the movie, *The Big Lebowski*, and loudly profess, "This aggression will not stand, man." Then I would get in my pickup truck and drive to Dr. Pilloni's chiropractic office for an adjustment. Why? Because getting checked and adjusted minimizes interference to your genetic potential AND hits a virtual reset button on the brain and nervous system. Notice how I didn't mention anything about going to the chiropractor for back pain? This from the guy who has had, many times severely so, back pain episodes beginning at age ten.

The latest research has established that the role of the chiropractic adjustment is to create input into the brain that acts as a reboot or reset button (I realize I am beating the hell out of the reset button analogy) to create the opportunity for the computer to restore balance. This is huge people. I always wondered why hardly any of my patients in twenty-five years of practice developed really serious life threatening health problems. Some did develop serious issues to be sure, but it was rare and the vast majority were significantly and profoundly healthier than the non-chiropractic humanity. Simply put, the brain runs the show but it gets stressed and getting adjusted re-sets the system, conferring measurable health benefits to people regardless of the presence or absence of pain or symptoms. (More information supplied in the appendix.)

The bottom line is just get adjusted by an awesome chiropractor anywhere from once/week to once/month for the rest of your long, fruitfully healthy life. A happy healthy brain and nervous system is the perfect complement to moving your body, putting good stuff in your gullet, and learning lots.

Caution: Yet another mountain analogy ahead.

I realize the previous description is complicated, so allow me to provide an example of genetic intelligence at work in my favorite sport of mountain climbing.

The Aconcagua of Health

I was planning my first attempt of Everest in 2007 but realized I needed more experience at high altitude beforehand. Therefore, I looked around and decided on an attempt of the highest mountain in the Western Hemisphere, Aconcagua, in 2006. The mountain sits on the Argentinian side of the Andes range, close to the early 1970's plane crash of the Uruguayan rugby team made famous in the book and movie *Alive* by Piers Paul Reade. An additional draw for me would be getting a crack at my third of the Seven Summits, or the highest mountain on each continent.

We started out at 7,000 feet, which is way higher than the fifty feet of elevation in Rhode Island where I live but doable if you drink a ton of water, eat a lot, and go slowly. Because of atmospheric pressure, there is more oxygen available to us closer to sea level and, as the climber gets higher in altitude, the oxygen molecules are farther apart and not as available to the body; hence, the need to acclimatize, which means taking a few days of slow ascent, like in Aconcagua, or a few weeks on a higher mountain, like Everest.

On any high mountain, like Kilimanjaro, Denali, Rainier, Everest, or Aconcagua, climbers will make higher camps and go lower to sleep in order for the body to acclimatize—climb high and sleep low. This facilitates the body's adaptation to the extreme physical, chemical, and emotional (yes, all three) stresses of hypoxia, or not enough oxygen.

The goal is to shock the body (stress) then let the innate bodily functions adapt to maintain life and survive.

If you do it right, you can ascend without getting acute mountain sickness, or AMS, or two of the primary high-altitude killer diseases, like brain swelling and lung swelling, known as HACE and HAPE, respectively. The human body has an incredible ability to adapt to stress, such as high altitude, if there is no interference in the nervous system.

You can read much more about mountaineering, and its life and death perils of body and mind, in my book, *Lessons from Everest: 7 Powerful Steps to the Top of Your World* (available on Amazon and Kindle).

Altitude sickness is no stroll in the park. I have been afflicted on many climbs around the world as I am a little slower to acclimatize initially than most of my teammates, but I rally and become stronger later in the expedition when it counts.

AMS feels not unlike being on a treadmill, jacked up to the max in speed and elevation, while breathing through a straw and having the worst influenza of your life while simultaneously experiencing the worst hangover of your life all without any energy, appetite or will to live for that matter. Combine all this with a headache like someone is pounding a railroad spike into your temple. Bad, bad, and doubly bad all at the same time.

In this sorry state, I did my best to remain upright at Aconcagua base camp at 15,000 feet, unable to think, move, or help do camp chores and, stating it here publicly for the first time, projectile vomiting my lunch with gusto in my teammate Big Tim Medvitz's tent site. Stay with me please. Believe it or not I am arriving at a point.

A day later, I was better. I took care of myself by resting and hydrating and forcing myself to eat. Several days later I summited the highest mountain in the Western Hemisphere and returned safely. My third of the famed Seven Summits. My genetic intelligence was doing its thing in response to the nearly overwhelming stress of oxygen deficit. Myriad chemical changes occurred inside and outside of the trillions of cells in my body. Respiration and cardiovascular adaptations happened, vast amounts of new red blood cells to efficiently carry oxygen molecules were put on a fast track of production in my bone marrow. Mini miracles all.

Thomas Edison et al.

The doctor of the future will give no medicine but will educate their patients in nutrition and the care of the human frame.
—Thomas A. Edison

That was written 125 years ago and is still true today. Additionally, to Edison's insight, I would have added care of the human mind. His message is more important than ever because it has been reported in 2016 that 31% of all Americans and 34% of American men are obese, up from 11% in 1975. Sure as shooting, this stopped me right in my tracks.

Do you mean to tell me that all the newspaper articles, TV news stories, public relations campaigns, government programs, hospitals, state and local organizations, gyms, trainers, biggest losers, Oprahs, Michelle Obamas, PSAs, MBAs, PhDs, thousands of books, late night infomercials, swimsuit editions, committees, subcommittees, and the associated billions of dollars have all been for naught, wasted? American bottoms are the biggest in history with all that money spent and all that attention?

I totally get that flab is not entirely the reason that we, Americans, are bringing up the rather large rear in regard to health and wellness in the developed world we inhabit, but morbidly obese Americans are certainly a daily observable symptom.

Don't believe me that the United States is unhealthy? We are way behind in many health categories. For example, according to the World Health Organization, America ranks 37th out of 190 in overall health, just ahead of Slovenia but behind Oman, which is #8; Morocco, which is #29; and Dominica, which is #35.

Let us look at just one heartbreaking example that has been just plain wrong for decades: Infant mortality. The fact that a child born in a big city hospital in Chicago has significantly less chance of survival (5.87 deaths per 1,000 live births) than a baby born in Cuba (4.63 deaths per 1,000 live births) according to the World Health Organization, is not only sorrowful but plain embarrassing.

The previous statistic has been true for decades, too, because I remember lecturing about the poor state of affairs in American health care thirty years ago, using infant mortality as the example.

The bad news is that we Americans are fat and unhealthy. The good news is that if we take responsibility for ourselves, our families, we can change it. We can become optimally well, and it's really not that hard. We can do it in one second by taking responsibility for ourselves, number one. We can do it in this instant, number two, by making just one healthy choice while not making an unhealthy one. Remember your virtual daily dashboard and ask constantly: "What would serve me now?" and "What do I need now?"

Number three, by making a healthy choice in ALL dimensions of Feet, Fork, and Fun—taking a walk, adding an extra vegetable per meal, and reading a book—our country and our world will shift on its axis. Our American bottoms will be smaller as well.

If I had to prescribe two things to improve health and happiness in the world it's movement and play.—Jason Nemer

The History of Stress

D. D. Palmer (1845-1913) was the first guy that I know of who wrote about the three facets of health, only he referred to Feet, Fork, and Fun as "the three T's: toxins, thoughts, and trauma." He was the founder of the profession of chiropractic in 1895—a brilliant thinker, writer, and practitioner of natural drug-free healing but also a lousy parent and a bit of a showboat.

Hans Selye, known by the unfortunate moniker of "the father of stress" (1907-1982), wrote in 1936 that chronic stress was a major cause of disease because of the predictable chemical changes that occur in an attempt to restore homeostasis, or internal balance. This theory became known as his "general adaptation syndrome," where Selye theorized that pressures, tensions, and other stressors greatly influence normal metabolism and that there was a limited supply of adaptive energy to deal with stress which declines with continuous exposure. Major bummer.

Every stress leaves an indelible scar, and the organism pays for its survival after a stressful situation by becoming a little older.
—Hans Selye

It would be significantly more of a major bummer if it was true, but thankfully it's not. I mention him because much of his "stress will kill you" misinformation is still actively promulgated in pop science and in the media today. Sure, runaway, unrelenting accumulating negative stresses involving the body, chemistry, and mind cause disease and dis-ease. Just not for the readers of this book who implement my simple admonitions.

Let's get clear about stress. There are good stresses and bad stresses. The goal of tone and Feet, Fork, and Fun is accumulating healthy good stresses and minimizing negative unhealthy stresses.

I have found that most people think all stress will kill them and eat them for dinner. The stress they are referring to is only one-sixth of stress and is the bad part of emotional stress. When this aspect of life, say a particularly frustrating coworker you have to deal with every day, is constant, you could feel a lack of control over the circumstance which can be particularly harmful. The result on the body over an extended time with this circumstance causes increased inflammation, weight gain, higher blood pressure and blood sugar, decreased immune and digestion functions, and the big ones: decreased sex hormone production and brain cell death. In this scenario, I can see where stress gets its bad rap but let's keep that mind open shall we?

You Mean Stress Heals?

Dr. Kelly McGonigal from Stanford University is a professor and the author of *The Upside of Stress*. In Dr. McGonigal's book, she reiterates the fact that you hear it all the time: stress causes heart disease, stress will give you a stroke, stress will prevent sleep which will kill you. In short, stress is bad, bad, bad and it's going to kill you, crash your car, and foreclose on your house—in that order.

What if, she posits, everything you thought you knew about stress was wrong, and what if changing your mind about stress could actually make you happier, more well, and better able to reach your goals and keep your house?

McGonigal offers an updated view on Selye's stress theory, one that reveals the good side of stress. Stress is not always harmful, and in many cases it makes us stronger, smarter, and happier. She even suggests that it can inspire compassion and enhance empathy, but how we feel about stress really makes a difference.

Rather than trying to escape stress as something to be avoided at all cost, I want you to embrace stress. The exercises, suggestions, and habits I put forth in this book are congruent with this suggestion. From Palmer to McGonigal, the understanding and usage of stress as wellness tool gradually became evident to me and is the backbone (Ha!) of the path to health and looking and feeling great.

OK. You say you got it about this stress thing, eh? The question remains, just how do we minimize negative accumulating stress in a complicated world? Answer: You buffer it! You buffer it with your new, shiny improved lifestyle. Examples of lifestyle buffers that accentuate coping skills and minimize the bad stress while enhancing your sense of well-being include: regular exercise of the correct type and timing, meditating/ mindfulness on a deep level with occasional deep cleansing breathes, renewing leisure activities you may have dropped along the way, increased care, feeding and time spent with your tribe(s), volunteering, doing something for others, contributing, and a few others like listening to music, being in nature, raising children wherever you find them, and reading and studying. The possibilities are limitless for good stresses overpowering bad.

Don't get overwhelmed or droopy eyed at this point as the proposed lifestyle of tone is easier to maintain than you may think. Go to www.drtimwarren.com and download the free "Week Sheet" to manage the magic.

Chapter Two: Brain Train Exercise

Daily Nervous System De-stress with Dr. Tim's Two-Minute Brain Wake Up Call

1. Cross crawl. Stand on one leg for fifteen seconds while bending slightly at the trunk while extending the opposite arm skyward. Do the other side.

2. Bullwinkle. Stand on a BOSU or folded towel for instability or just stand on your highest tippy-toes while with your thumbs massaging the indentations behind your ears simultaneously. Thirty seconds.

3. Hitchhike to Heaven. Stand with arms outstretched to the side, thumbs up, and while looking up squeeze shoulder blades together while moving arms in small circles. Thirty seconds.

4. Bad Wedding Dance. A gentle channeling of the Chubby Checker Twist using lumbar, back, and neck gently in motion. NOTE: These are demonstrated on my website.

The Zen of Tone

I have been so lucky to have spent time with native Sherpa and Nepalese people since 2007, including the month I spent hiking to Everest base camp with my teenage son after I pulled him from his senior year of high school.

Nepal is the world's sixth poorest country in addition to having the highest mountain. Two of the world's major religions are practiced there, Buddhism and Hinduism. It's always inspired me that religious devotees stand literally shoulder to shoulder worshiping in their own particular way in complete acceptance and peacefulness.

I have spent a fair amount of time with friends who are devoutly Buddhist and have observed their ritual worship on many occasions. It never fails to fascinate me how complicated and expensive (relative to their income) their devotions are. Many spend all day, almost like a second and third job, spinning prayer wheels, painting and installing prayer flags or wind horses, worshiping multiple deities, and purchasing kits of supplies daily to garner themselves in better stead with the creator or creators. As usual in religion, groups splinter off and go a different way. In contrast to the above complicated worship format, Zen Buddhism's followers eschew the pomp and ceremony and favor a simplified asceticism without the hullaballoo.

Here's the point: implementation of a health development lifestyle has similarities to complicated religions. For many people, getting and staying healthy can appear just as complicated, expensive, time consuming, and possibly inconsequential. Healthy living does not and should not be as complicated or take up huge swathes of time like a highly ritualized religion. We make healthy living so much harder than it has to be. Don't overthink and underdo. Change a habit today that no longer serves you. Add a good and subtract a bad. Keep doing good stuff and stop doing bad stuff. It's as simple as that. Live these adages simply and persistently. Stay tuned.

Chapter Two: Points to Ponder

1. Your health is a "mountain" of balance in three dimensions Feet, Fork, and Fun.
2. Tone is the vision or purpose of high vibrational living in the above three dimensions.
3. Your brain needs rebooting occasionally.
4. Your body self-heals better if it is not interfered with.
5. Stress is not necessarily bad despite what the media professes.
6. Increase good stress and decrease bad stress.
7. Making good, healthy, high vibrational choices is easier than you think.
8. Get checked and adjusted regularly by a chiropractor. Not sure who to go to? See the appendix.
9. De-stress your spine, body, and brain with Dr. Tim's Two-Minute Brain Wake-up Call. For every hour of sitting (office, car, TV, Red Sox game) do an extra set.

CHAPTER THREE

Have a Nice Decay

People Don't Die, They Kill Themselves Slowly.
—Patrick Gentempo, DC

Decay Happens

Decay happens with disuse. An empty house deteriorates at a significantly faster rate than a house that people live in. Airplanes that are grounded disintegrate at a significantly faster rate.

People are absolutely the same way. People who are inactive, who do not move, deteriorate at a way higher and faster level than people who are active. Humans are created to move and if we don't we die, slowly perhaps, but we die nonetheless.

A recent study of 2,600 Americans who wore sensors was not encouraging. We are on our butts and barely moving. Obese women averaged eleven seconds/day of vigorous exercise while normal weight men and women were vigorous (on the level of a jog or brisk uphill hike) for less than two minutes per day according to the *Mayo Clinic Proceedings*. Edward Archer, the nutrition and obesity lead author at the University of Alabama Birmingham determined, "How you spend your day determines whether you store your food as fat or store your food in your muscle, healthfully."

Nature is always in motion. If you look through an electron microscope at the inner workings of, say, a human skin cell or a pomegranate cell, stuff is moving and shaking. Objects are moving around inside a cell, nothing is stationary. If you look even deeper than that, down to the subatomic particles, things are flying around at breakneck speed. The building blocks of molecules and life are zipping around energetically and yet we get up in the morning, sit, get in the car for work or school and sit, drive home and sit in front of the TV, then get up and do the same thing all over again. Then one day sooner or later we don't get up. Are you sold yet on the importance of moving?

Our bodies, made up of 70 trillion cells and an incalculable number of tinier objects, have to move and have proper nutrition in order to function well. Lifestyle diseases exist because of not moving, eating, and thinking well—the opposite of toned paying-attention-to-the-moment living.

Back to brain health for a moment, Dr. Roger Sperry, Nobel-winning brain researcher, found that movement of the spine is like a "windmill generator to the brain and nervous system" and the "sensory stimulation to the brain was like a nutritional pump directly to the brain." Sperry also determined that "90% of the stimulation to the brain comes from movement of the spine." Hey all, the brain is like a muscle and needs to be exercised and when we exercise the body, the brain gets exercised! Cool. Saves time that way. By the way did I mention that everybody who owns a spine should go to the chiropractor regularly for brain exercise? And, do the daily Dr. Tim's brain wake-up call activities as often each day as possible.

Lifestyle chronic diseases are the leading cause of death and disability in the United States today and can be prevented or minimized significantly with the common sense healthy lifestyle espoused within these pages. Chronic diseases and conditions include heart disease, stroke, cancer, type 2 diabetes, obesity, and arthritis—the most common, costly, and preventable of all health problems.

As of 2012, according to the U.S. Centers for Disease Control and Prevention, about half of all adults, or 117 million people, had one or more chronic health conditions. One of four adults had two or more chronic health conditions. Seven of the top ten causes of death were chronic diseases. Two of these chronic diseases—heart disease and cancer—together accounted for nearly 48% of all deaths.

Obesity is a serious health concern. During 2009 to 2010, more than one-third of adults, or about 78 million people, were obese. Nearly one of five youths aged 2 to 19 years was obese with a BMI (body mass index) above the 95th percentile.

Arthritis is the most common cause of disability. Of the 53 million adults with doctor-diagnosis arthritis, more than 22 million say they have trouble with their usual activities because of arthritis.

Diabetes is the leading cause of kidney failure, lower limb amputations other than those caused by injury, and new cases of blindness among adults.

Health risk behaviors are unhealthy behaviors you can change. Four of these health risk behaviors—lack of exercise or physical activity, poor nutrition, tobacco use, and drinking too much alcohol—cause much of the illness, suffering, and early death related to chronic diseases and conditions.

In 2011, more than half (52%) of adults age 18 and older did not meet recommendations for aerobic exercise or physical activity. In addition, 76% did not meet recommendations for muscle-strengthening physical activity.

About half of American adults (47%) have at least one of the following major risk factors for heart disease or stroke: uncontrolled high blood pressure, uncontrolled high LDL cholesterol (the bad cholesterol), or are current smokers. About 90% of Americans consume too much salt, increasing their risk of high blood pressure.

In 2011, more than one-third (36%) of adolescents and 38% of adults said they ate fruit less than once a day, while 38% of adolescents and 23% of adults say they ate vegetables less than once a day.

More than 42 million adults, close to one of every five, said they currently smoked cigarettes in 2012. Cigarette smoking accounts for more than 480,000 deaths each year. Each day, more than 3,200 youths younger than 18 years smoke their first cigarette, and another 2,100 youths and young adults who smoke every now and then later become daily smokers.

Drinking too much alcohol is responsible for 88,000 deaths each year, more than half of which are due to binge drinking. About 38,000 American adults report binge drinking an average of four times a month, who have an average of eight drinks per binge, yet most binge drinkers are not alcohol dependent.

The Cost of Chronics

In the United States, chronic diseases and conditions and the health risk behaviors that cause them account for most health care costs, and 86% of all health care spending in 2010 was for people with one or more chronic medical conditions. The total cost of heart disease and stroke in 2010 was estimated to be $315.4 billion. Of this amount, $193.4 billion was for direct medical costs, not including costs of nursing home care.

Cancer care cost $157 billion in 2010. The total estimated cost of diagnosed diabetes in 2012 was $245 billion, including $176 billion in direct medical costs and $69 billion in decreased productivity.

Let me stop here and remind readers of the two most important questions to ask yourself throughout your day, not shouted out loud perhaps, but to yourself: "What do I need right now?" and "What would serve me best right now?"

Decreased productivity includes costs associated with people being absent from work, being less productive while at work, or not being able to work at all because of diabetes.

The total cost of arthritis and related conditions was about $128 billion in 2003 (most definitely way more in today's dollars). Of this amount, nearly $81 billion was for direct medical costs, and $47 billion was for indirect costs associated with lost earnings.

Medical costs linked to obesity were estimated to be $147 billion in 2008. Annual medical costs for people who are obese were $1,429 higher per person than for those people of normal weight in 2006.

For the years between 2009 and 2012, economic costs due to smoking were estimated to be more than $289 billion a year. This cost includes at least $133 billion in direct medical care for adults and more than $156 billion for lost productivity from premature death estimated from 2005 to 2009.

Last, but not least, the economic costs of drinking too much alcohol were estimated to be $223.5 billion, or $1.90 per drink, in 2006. Most of these costs were due to binge drinking and resulted from losses in workplace productivity, health care expenses, and crimes related to excessive drinking.

GET BACK—The Beatles

Lowly back pain, experienced by eighty percent of people at some point or another, and near and dear to my heart—it was the reason I got into my profession allowing me to positively influence many thousands of people over twenty-five years—was also the reason I was forced to leave the profession because my back was killing me and preventing me from bending over to care for my patients.

If you remember the beginning of the book, I first went to a chiropractor at age nineteen because of leg and knee pain, numbness, and tingling, but the cause was chronic lower back dysfunction and dis-ease. My back exhibited no symptoms but I had compression in my lower back resulting in compression of the sciatic nerves, which are the largest nerves in the body supplying the legs.

Second only to the common cold as a reason for doctor's visits as well as second in missed work days, back pain results in a $50 billion price tag for our country, and is largely preventable. Just as with the lifestyle diseases previously mentioned, the vast majority of back pain cases, 80% to 90%, would be preventable if people lived toned.

Not counted in the $50 billion costs of back pain is the unfolding tragedy of addiction to pain killers, much of which started as an opioid prescription for a joint-related issue. Many became heroin addicted as a result and many have died, mostly started by being legally prescribed a narcotic, which opened Pandora's Box, kind of like a modern-day Dr. Frankenstein.

Keep on the lookout for my upcoming book, *Bad Back, Awesome Life*, in 2018.

Drugs, surgery, and hospitals are rarely the answer to chronic disease. Facilitating the God-given healing capacity that all of us have is key. Improved diet, exercise, and lifestyle is basic.
—Dr. Joe Mercola

Save America $1 Trillion (Dr. Tim Gets a Presidential Medal of Freedom)

It is easy to get lost in all these statistics and all these billions of dollars, but when you think about the cost just to our country of arthritis, type 2 diabetes, colds, flus, viruses (our immune function is also very much affected by lifestyle choices), heart disease, stroke, cancer, asthma, remember that all of these are affected by the way you live your life. Meaning, if your lifestyle gets healthier, the disease is either minimized, eliminated, or prevented—great for you and an unbelievable saving for us all—a classic win-win.

If you tally up all this stuff, it is easy to see how a trillion dollars could be saved if Americans truly took responsibility and worked every day to live toned. All I am asking for that $1 trillion saved is a measly little amount. Say 10%? Is that fair? On the other hand, I would gladly trade the $100,000,000,000 for that Medal of Freedom. Fair dinkum?

Health Armageddon

Go to the mall one day and sit with a coffee and do some people-watching. Don't be creepy about it, but just watch. What do you see? How many overweight children do you see? How about pathologically overweight entire families? How many people are limping? How many people have distorted shoulder heights? How many young people are using a cane? How many are in wheelchairs? How many pairs of eyes exhibit dullness? How many have poor skin or are muffin topped? And those are just what can be observed with clothes on.

I am always amazed by the sheer numbers of fixable health conditions being allowed to flourish by smart people not taking responsibility for their health and allowing their most precious possession to deteriorate without a fight. Change yourself and your family and you officially are doing your part. Not only for immediate loved ones but the U.S. of A and the world by being part of the solution while not participating in the cause.

If we do not act individually, we are going to go over the brink financial-wise, health-wise, and economic development-wise, resulting in a diminished standing in the world. One disease I will use as an example: Type 2 diabetes. Today pre-diabetes affects 86 million Americans. That's one in three of us according to the American Diabetes Association. This means all 86 million are probably headed for type 2 and a future of heart disease and stroke. Can you imagine the price tag? Can you imagine the individual and family suffering? Remember this is just one of the many lifestyle diseases. I am afraid that if today's disease trend continues there will be a new "Fall of the Roman Empire" without one bomb being dropped. I am not exaggerating. Do you think the cavalry in the form of the medical establishment will come to the rescue?

"Medical errors are now the number three cause of death in the United States." —British Medical Journal

There are a number of problems that demand attention in the world, I get it, but the disease care price tag will be fatal. That bill will come due in the next ten to twenty years if we don't change. Let's put the problem in a different non-economic perspective: the millennials of today will be the first generation to not outlive their parents. What is so frustrating is that it's preventable. Let's all simply cut the horrid lifestyle habits and get super-fit.

"Make America healthy again." —The Author

The Funky Future of Health Care

Are you a health optimist or a death pessimist? Do you think we will be thinner, fitter, and healthier ten years from now or chubbier, sicker, and on life-support ten years from now? I choose "tonier" despite my doom and gloom of the previous paragraphs.

Based on research, observations, and my genius insight, here are a few advances of thought and practice I see coming down the pike in health and wellness in our world. Most items are currently in active practice but will rise in utilization rates or become "viral" and commonplace. In other words, I see good stuff happening in the future.

1. People will accept that lifestyle—how they live their lives—is the best thing they can do for immunity and health. One example is that the use of antibiotics for routine minor issues will be a thing of the past. We have to learn to live with the buglets and microscopic creepy crawlies because they grow exponentially quicker than we can produce antibiotics to kill them. Plus, we need bugs in order to exist. Is that a good enough reason for you? This has been known for many decades but for one reason or another (profits for drug companies and laziness by doctors are two reasons) has not been understood by the masses. The classic germ theory of disease—that is, germs are the cause of us being sick and that if we do not come into contact with germs or if we kill the germs then we are going to be healthier—is a lie. The germ theory of disease started with Professor Robert Koch in

the late 1850s. This washed up BS is going to die a necessary death. If the germ theory of disease were true—that if a healthy person comes in contact with a germ he/she is going to get an illness—everybody would be dead. There would be nobody left to believe the theory. It is the health of the person not the virulence of the germ that determines if someone is going to get sick or not.

Not all people who are exposed to the HIV virus get infected. Not everybody in the same school, workplace, or family unit gets sick even though all are exposed to the same germs. Why? Because some people's immune systems were doing their job. Healthy people don't get sick, only sick people (read: diminished immune system) get sick.

Every day, we come into contact with kajillions of germs, many of which could kill us, but our own built-in resistance and our natural immunity modulated by our genetic intelligence takes care of business as long as the nervous system is not interfered with. When I get sick, and it's a rare event thankfully, it's my own damn fault. I was either burning the candle at both ends, eating poorly, or negatively stressed—in short, not toned.

2. Let's talk gut-brain connection, otherwise known as the microbiome. The digestive tract, the naturally occurring flora and fauna that live happily there, and the nervous system connections will be a major focus in health understanding for researchers and rank and file Americans. The gut-brain connection is a major part of our immune function and research being done right now is very exciting. One development, fecal transplants, is when a healthy person donates some of their fecal matter which is then used as a treatment for immune deficiency diseases such as *C. diff (Clostridium difficile)*. This common condition is an antibiotic-resistant hospital-borne infection that deteriorates the immune system. It wastes people. When people receive fecal transplants there is very close to a 90% cure rate in C. diff patients, naturally, with no side effects, no drugs, and a price tag of hundreds rather than tens of thousands. Thanks to my son Kurt, a biology researcher specializing in the microbiome, for exercising my understanding of this cutting edge science. This is the dawn of understanding of the relationship between fitness/health, our gut-brain axis, and natural immunity.

3. Increasingly, prescription drugs of all kinds will be minimized. They will be utilized a fraction of what they are now. We all see on TV or read in a magazine or newspaper advertisement every day about this or that wonderful drug that is going to cure humanity of a particular condition. A little while later, it is taken off the market because people who took it grew an extra ear, their forehead turned blue, they started listening to the Bay City Rollers, or they just died then and there. I jest but you and I have seen it multiple times. I am not saying that all drugs are bad at all times, but minimizing and curtailing the vast majority of those chemicals coming in contact with our chemistry is wise thinking. After all there is little science in the drug business. Everybody has different internal chemistries and it's a crap shoot as to what happens when you add a chemical cocktail into the naturally occurring body chemistry.

4. Minimizing any manner of chemical contact is part of the future of health care. Yard chemicals, household cleaning agents and solvents, personal grooming products, worksite substances, whatever—just be prudent about what you and your family come in contact with. Our air and water quality is another concern. I am very lucky to have awesome, tested, delicious well water from an environment that I can control. Pay attention to yours as best you can.

5. In the not-too-distant future, people are going to become more aware of the vitalistic nature of health and biological forces. All living things are sustained by a vital force, previously referred to as genetic potential or intelligence, a life force that is both different from and greater than physical and chemical forces. Genetic intelligence operates outside of currently known physical laws of the universe and self-heals us and self-regulates us without us even paying attention.

We simply do not know everything there is to know about this vital force, but we have an innate power to heal from the inside out, and as more people realize they possess this incredible power I am confident they will treat themselves better. When one understands there is a power within them that is doing everything it can to survive and thrive, improved self-care will be a big duh.

6. There is much we do not understand about the brain function, but in the future, we will have more insight. For example, with all the money and research that has been done, we still have no idea what a thought is. It seems like such a simple thing that happens kabillions of times every day, but scientists have no clue what a thought is and how it works. Is it chemical? Is it neural? Is it electrical? Is it God? Is it a combination? Nobody knows so we need to stick around for this one.

The brain and the spinal cord, known as the central nervous system, control and coordinate all functions and parts of the body by utilizing the nerves (peripheral nervous system) of the body like telephone wires.

7. Inflammation: one of the few universally agreed upon causes of lifestyle dis-ease is inflammation. Inflammation and how our lifestyle choices minimize it will be universally understood in tomorrow's family health plan. Today, experts say chronic inflammation plays a role in eleven of the top fifteen causes of death in the United States. The importance of having a low inflammation lifestyle is one of the few concepts in health that is generally accepted by doctors and researchers of all stripes today. Inflammation leads to the lifestyle diseases previously noted and proper exercise and, most assuredly, proper nutrition help reduce inflammation and, therefore, will reduce those chronic diseases that are the leading causes of death, disability, and expense in the developed world. Note: the Feet, Fork, and Fun lifestyle and protocol in Part II are instrumental in lowering inflammation.

8. I believe that all dairy and all meats will be from only grass-fed and free-range animals. This rapid changeover is happening already as I am sure you have noticed. I don't recommend dairy products traditionally produced, but would give the OK to hormone-free, drug-free, cage-free, grass-fed, non-chemically adulterated products.

In the future the vast majority of our vegetables will either be grown at home or purchased from a nearby farmer's market, and all will be organic. I was lucky enough to grow up in a household sporting a large vegetable garden and, in addition to the dog, cats, and horses, each of us three kids had at different times our own beef animal. Mine was Rodney. Rodney eventually became the best tasting hamburger that I have experienced to this day. Although I whined incessantly about my garden and livestock chores (including having to milk the one milk cow by hand before school), all the veggies were organic and the meat was grass-fed before we were even familiar with the terms.

As far as genetically modified organisms (GMO) are concerned, for me the jury is still out on this. I have not seen anything that leads me to believe that it is as bad as some claim, however, in the future our understanding of genetically modified organisms will be manifest.

The closer we can emulate our food procurement and activity levels to that of the hunter-gatherer, the closer we come to living as our nature intended. The result being the human race will become the best version of itself.

Chapter Three: Brain Train Exercise—Super Brain Yoga

Super brain yoga doesn't involve any strange bodily contortions, is simple to perform, and is a beneficial stimulating brain exercise. I would recommend it to parents of ADD/ADHD children, senile or autistic people, not to mention everyone who wants a sharper mind for life—from an investment of two to five minutes per day. Try for fourteen slow repetitions.

1. Face east, remove any jewelry, and press your tongue firmly on the roof of your mouth.

2. With left arm first, reach over and grasp right earlobe with thumb on the outside and two fingers on the inside.

3. Do the same with your right arm.

4. Inhale deeply through your nose while simultaneously squatting to a sitting position. Extra credit if you can go down almost to floor level. Hold for two to three seconds, if possible.

5. This is one rep. Inhale down and exhale up. Continue for fourteen reps/day.

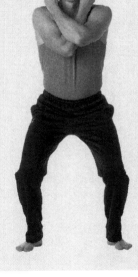

Money, money, money, money mo-ney! —The O'Jays

Why do you think the federal government's Food Guide Pyramid and its newest incarnation My Plate (www.myplate.gov), is the way that it is? Do you think it's because the United States government wants us to be as healthy as possible or because big money corrupted the process? Let's look at the nutrition pyramid by the USDA.

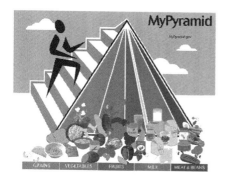 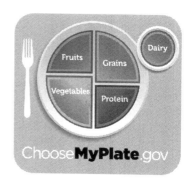

As the reader has undoubtedly noted, I like mountain shapes of all kinds... except for the USDA Food Pyramid. I dislike this triangle intensely. In fact, it gives me agita. I believe this U.S. Department of Agriculture/U.S. Department of Health and Human Services program robs the American public of the truth about nutritional health and furthermore robs them of their health and deteriorates their bodies through inflammation. It's appalling that the diagram is put in front of the public by the very federal bureaucracies that have been entrusted to give us valid health information. Why? All I can fathom is money. Big Agriculture has deep pockets for lobbying efforts. Some companies don't want to lose money even if it means not being entirely truthful to the public. Alternatively, here is my nutritional mountain.

You may think the differences between disease, wellness, and super-wellness are relatively obvious but take a look-see at the Chapter Ten Brain Train Exercise to explore more fully.

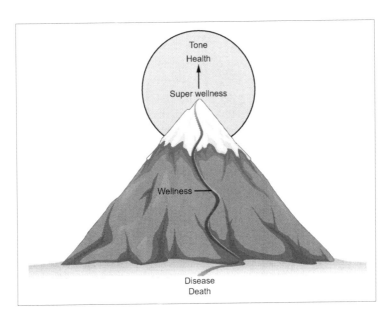

Fallacy and Foolishness in the Food Pyramid

Do you think a bowl of Frosted Flakes is healthier than an avocado? Your federal government does. Your taxes paid for this nugget of health misinformation that the average four-year-old would shake her head at. Do you think the recently retired food pyramid, which has morphed into MyPlate.gov, is a Big Agriculture, money-driven, lobby-fest sham resulting in embarrassingly poor health recommendations? Can you believe our tax dollars entrusted to the federal government to tell the truth have been hijacked by the underbelly of big business? You be the judge after reading Chapter Seven but, as a teaser for Chapter Seven, Fork, here is Dr. Tim's Plate.

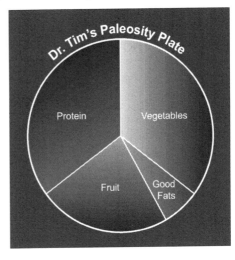

Why Smart People Make Dumb Health Decisions

We all have our own "stuff" that we either choose to deal with or not. Too many people feel that fitness or health is something they can put off in the short term and deal with later. After all, there are some items that are more pressing at the moment such as living from one crisis to another and carving out a rut of complacency, rationalization, apathy, and procrastination. Please don't get in a health and wellness C.R.A.P. rut. After all, we heard somewhere that a rut has something to do with a coffin with the ends knocked out. The solution: start now.

Chapter Three: Points to Ponder

1. Motion = Life. Motion = life both microscopically and macroscopically.

2. Americans are not generally healthy and the trends are worsening.

3. People unwittingly kill themselves slowly.

4. If you get a cold, it's your fault, not the virus's or a nearby person who also has low internal resistance and got ill.

5. All doctors surprisingly agree that inflammation kills many and is lifestyle-related and therefore preventable.

6. Take responsibility for your inflammation by following the Feet, Fork, and Fun protocol in Part Two.

CHAPTER FOUR

Feet, Fork, and Fun

Do what you can, with what you have, where you are.
—Theodore Roosevelt

Stress Me Bro

Still think stress is bad? Dr. McGonigal in her book, *The Upside of Stress*, refutes the "father of stress," Hans Selye, and gives credence to philosopher, Friedrich Nietzsche's oft-quoted quip, "that which doesn't kill me makes me stronger."

Please note I am not suggesting trauma as stress—just good old-fashioned hardship occasionally, and research shows that hardship and the resulting resiliency that inevitably follows makes us stronger.

For example, bacteria that are not killed entirely by an antibiotic (stress) often mutate and become resistant to antibiotics (gain strength). People who start a sane exercise program from scratch (stress) will quickly improve their fitness (resiliency).

McGonigal further makes the point that emotional stress from a hardship can inspire compassion and inspire empathy. After major calamities (stress) thousands stand in line to give blood and support each other (strength). Have you noticed this in your life?

Several years ago when I was going through a divorce and experiencing negative psychological stress, I felt significantly more empathy with my patients I was caring for and felt like I did the best doctoring of my career. What if I said you would die without stress? You would, and we all would. We need stress to survive and thrive.

A sometimes confusing concept to understand is that of good stress versus bad stress in the three human dimensions of physical, chemical, and emotional. Please allow me to illustrate the difference using an example of experiences I had at Ground Zero in New York City in the aftermath of the 9/11 tragedy.

Ground Zero

In September 2001, just days after the towers fell, a call went out for chiropractors to staff two twenty-four-hour chiropractic clinics within Ground Zero proper to care for the workers there. My Rhode Island colleague Dr. Robitaille and I couldn't get there quick enough. We were credentialed by the American Red Cross and settled in, adjusting construction workers, police, national guard members, and fellow volunteers.

The first negative I noticed was chemical. Upon entrance to Ground Zero we were sprayed down with what I presumed was an antibiotic fluid, especially our feet. The chemical debris scent of Ground Zero was most distinctive and found later to be highly toxic. All manner of yucky was in that air space from asbestos to jet fuel to... I don't really want to know what else.

More than 1,100 Ground Zero workers have been diagnosed with cancer since 9/11. The closest I can describe the stench was when I fell asleep once boiling a can of sweetened condensed milk in my home in order to make caramel. Of course I promptly fell asleep and the can later exploded, coating my kitchen floor to ceiling with burnt sugary goo. That burnt sugary goo smelled almost exactly like the carcinogenic air at Ground Zero. Negative stress in the chemical dimension.

There were extensive examples of negative physical stress from Ground Zero including the small army of construction specialists doing what they called "working the pile." Untold hours on and off heavy equipment. At this time in October, work was still above the ground, and they were removing steel girders that were glowing white hot from underground pressure. Negative stress in the physical dimension.

As a country we had no idea if more attacks were imminent, and even if they weren't, Americans everywhere realized that life as we knew it before 9/11 was gone forever. Those working inside Ground Zero were surrounded by death, uncertainty, sadness, and awe at the enormity of it all. Negative psychological stress in the emotional dimension.

At dinner, I observed a construction worker who was obviously struggling to hold it together. The man sat alone and though stoic was obviously cracking at the seams. It was then that a Red Cross manager on the lookout for just such situations sat down with the man and spoke to him as if they were ensconced in a down home Iowa coffee shop.

I watched as the man visibly unwound and calmed.

Most people, if asked to define stress, would relate the common negative aspects of emotional stress, which is actually only one-sixth of stress.

Three Dimensions and Three Cures

My math may be a bit off but bear with me. In my earth-shattering Nobel-worthy $3 \times 3 \times 3 = 6$-pack formula, the first three stands for the three dimensions of human health: The physical, the chemical, and the emotional—or Feet, Fork, and Fun.

The second 3 is our goal of increasing, embracing, or facilitating positive stress in those three dimensions. For example, doing Dr. Tim's one-second exercises is positive stress in the Feet realm, adding more good quality protein is a good development in the Fork realm, and reviewing your 3×5 intention card first thing in the morning after making your bed is a great development in the Fun component.

The third 3 means minimizing, through our lifestyle choices, the negative aspects of those three stresses. For example, minimizing sitting is an example of lessened negative stress in the Feet area, having two or less sugary desserts/week is minimizing stress in the Fork dimension, and the fact that you spent time reading this awesome inspiring new book (and didn't listen to bombastic yelling and screaming hyperbolic talk radio on the way to work this morning) lessens stress in the psychological or Fun arena.

Putting it all together, our first job is to be aware of potentially good and bad stresses, activities, or habits. Next, we accentuate the positive stresses and minimize the negative stresses. It's that simple. Perfection only exists in nature so don't add negative psychological stress by aiming for that which is unattainable. After all it's what you do most of the time that counts.

Chapter Four: Brain Train Exercise— Ten Weird Health Tips in Three Dimensions

Throw a party: social connections help you live longer. (Fun Dimension)

Adopt a pet: pets lead to healthier hearts and lowered blood pressure. (Fun)

Have some dark chocolate, at least 70% cacao. (Fork)

Grind your own black organic coffee. (Fork)

Have two glasses or less of wine. (Fork)

Have sex as it helps the brain, improves immunity, and lowers depression risk. (Feet and Fun)

Listen to your fave tunes. (Fun)

Take a nap. (Feet, Fork, and Fun)

Get outdoors and breathe good air. (Feet, Fun)

Stay away from chemicals, especially antibacterial products. (Fork)

You Have a Six-Pack Right Now

Why six-pack as the goal or result? Six-pack is a euphemism of tone. I am not making the case that your idea of tone should even include traditional six-pack abdominals. I don't have them. Let me rephrase that: We all have a six-pack, it's just that in the vast majority of humans they aren't visible behind a layer of adipose tissue. You can certainly live toned without a visible six-pack so it remains for you to decide. For many years I sported a "visible" six-pack and was relatively proud of it but now I find it's not on my goal list. A key tidbit of information was the realization that you can be perfectly healthy without the adornment of bumps on your core. It is too hard to achieve and maintain for me so I would relegate the care and feeding of a visible six-pack as significant negative stress in my psychological, chemical, and physical dimensions. Your tone is your business and is defined by your intentions and desires. I personally wouldn't waste time and effort by having a six-pack abdomen goal—or any health goal based on appearances. A bigger vision is energy, wellness, health, minimizing disease if present, preventing future disease if possible, and Fun, Fun, Fun. Is it your dream to worry and fret about the gain and loss of two pounds? I would wager only if you are paid fat stacks as a cover model.

Great News Alert

I have the most awesome news for you, my svelte and buff reader. This news is so shockingly great that I can barely contain myself to jot it down in my MacBook. I am frozen in near ecstasy with the importance of sharing this garnish of fantastic news with you, the student of tone. I could go on here and really overdo it but will force myself to get on with it. Allow me a drum roll please? Thanks!

Ok. The awesome-sauce news is this: When you make ANY positive change in ANY of the three dimensions OR eliminate a negative in any of the three dimensions, second drum roll please, ALL of the dimensions improve. Everything improves! For example, if you begin an exercise program (positive physical dimension) the Fork and Fun dimensions are also positively enhanced. If you positively change your chemical dimension by, say, adding another vegetable serving/day or eliminating fried food, your Feet AND Fun arenas are rockin' and rollin' as well. Lastly, if all you accomplished was setting some personal goals that you deeply care about and putting them on your intention card (positive emotional dimension) your Feet and Fork function (say that three times fast) will be poised to skyrocket.

Even if you only improve one positive stress or minimize one negative stress in only one dimension, your overall vibration and wellness are greatly improved and primed for a real personal health revolution and breakthrough. Hopefully this realization alone will remove permanently the health guilt and overwhelm that plagues so many Americans and stymies them from achieving the health, fitness, and tone that they and their families deserve.

Ask Dr. Tim if Getting Off Your Butt Is Right for You

Who is the CEO of you? That would be you so add the initials and title to your name from now on. Remember that taking responsibility for everything is the first admonition in an important, success philosopher's famous book? Never forget that you are the boss of you. Also, never forget that most of success in life is showing up. Showing up means starting your climb of Mount Tone right now, where you stand. Really. I mean right now. Make a decision that honors your genetic intelligence. Instantly do or change or add something right now. You have digested enough of this book, no pun intended, to begin a transformation or revolution in your life so be the CEO and start now. Can't think of a worthy item to add or subtract? Is there somebody you need to contact? Is there something you really should have done yesterday and it's bugging you? Do it now. What you receive is minimized negative stress and a bump in overall vibration and tone.

You may not want to share with anybody your intention for tone. Do not confide in the peeps who will not support you 100% in your striving to climb your mountain. Better yet, just start, then observe how soon people notice your personal revolution. They may see it in your face first. Excitement, zest, and commitment will be evident in your face and eyes before any discernible morphological change is observable. In my experience with 250,000 patients and clients, the ones who were truly serious about personal improvement had truly revolutionary positive changes within two weeks. What they may be for you I don't know but it will be Fun, Fun, Fun.

Accept graciously and humbly all compliments and quizzical looks that come your way and keep on keeping on. If folks ask what you are doing to look so energetic and focused feel free to refer them to my website www.drtimwarren.com and suggest they spend great gobs of money there so they summit Mount Tone as well. After all, don't forget my goal of pocketing 10% of the trillion dollars that I save the United States in future health care costs or receiving a Medal of Freedom or preferably both. You, my sexy friend, are on a wondrous never ending quest to harness and achieve your human potential—the best you, you can be. This fabulous journey should be continued until you are 120 years old then maybe you can take a day off or add a third cheat meal per week. Your choice.

What is now proved was once only imagined.
—William Blake

It doesn't really matter where your health starting point is. If you are a quadriplegic in a wheelchair, there is much you can do to ramp up (again no pun intended) your wellness. Two-thirds of positive stress, fork and fun—or chemical and emotional—is available for maximizing human potential. We must also never underestimate developments in technology and understanding that will inevitably occur. Never lose hope regardless of the situation and remember to take responsibility and concentrate on what you can do in the moment, not what you can't.

Please don't fall into victim mentality. I'm not saying that in the past you have not been victimized and I am definitely not saying "get over it." However, some can benefit from moving on from the victim mindset. How would you know if you may be playing the victim card? A. Blaming other people and circumstances. B. Feeling righteous in a disagreement. C. Breaking promises and agreements chronically. If any or all of these describe you, snap out of it! Instead, try: A. In a problem or disagreement observe your contribution. B. Honor commitments. C. Pay more attention to your own actions and accountability than other people's.

No Discipline? No Sweat.

What's that you say? No discipline? Stop saying that please. It's one of those whatcha-call-it self-fulfilling prophesies! Shut up about it and start living. Get used to the great feelings that permeate your soul when you do repeated positive things for body and mind. Doing anything will change the dynamics, but you must be on guard for C.R.A.P. (as a reminder, Complacency, Rationalization, Apathy, and Procrastination). Remember that even if you maximize one measly positive stress and minimize one tiny picayune negative, you have changed fundamentally your personal operating system. Continue updating your personal operating system till you're 120.

In Chapter Ten, The Everest 70 Challenge, you will learn the easy, doable, focused plan for updating your operating system in the moment to achieve a real, deeply rewarding healthy lifestyle.

The more relaxed you are the better you are at everything.
—Bill Murray

Achieving Peak Energy

Are you a high energy, project-accomplishing dynamo? Personally, I love having the energy to live the life I want. If I don't have energy during the day, then I ask myself if I need a water or snack break or I'll grab a ten-minute power nap. It's a binary function really. A big Yes to this or that which moves me up the fitness/health continuum and a resounding No to that which moves me down. The funny thing about having energy is you have to expend it to get it. This is counterintuitive for some. Moving your body, improving your nutrition, learning things, harnessing the power of your mindset get you highly energetic and ready for more accomplishment. Energy begets energy and fun begets fun. Resting and recuperating are greatly enhanced and the lowly under appreciated nap becomes an adventure in luxurious living. Note: I have found that the best naps are between ten and thirty minutes and are best flat on a carpet with no pillow. Eyeshade is ok. I find these quick-hit naps offer energy-boosting benefits without any droopiness afterward.

Fartlek for Feet, Fork, and Fun

Fartlek, besides being a hilarious word to sprinkle liberally into conversation in polite company, is an important tenet of Feet, Fork, and Fun. The word fartlek is a Swedish term roughly translating to "speed play." Fartlek accentuates the health-enhancing stresses of fitness and minimizes the detrimental.

I first learned the technique of fartlek while researching running physiology in junior high school cross country. We trained on hill and dale using various speeds—fast, slow, and medium (sometimes we started off slow then tapered off)—up hills and down to enhance our chances of crushing our schoolboy rivals in weekly two- to three-mile races. Decades later, even if it's not called fartlek, the principles of varying the exercise stress in sport and fitness training is ubiquitous. Not a competitive athlete you say? I beg to differ. I believe that we are all athletes, inner and outer, and we all have one large looming, sometimes cantankerous adversary: ourselves. Don't compete against anyone but yourself if you choose but remember there is no greater competition than the one against the person in the mirror.

The human body has an incredible ability to adapt. The body quickly gets used to the positive stress of exercise and then hard work becomes less fruitful though certainly not useless. The fix is shaking it up. Do different activities and sequences. What you usually do first now do last. Shake it up with fartlek. Feel free to insert chuckling here. The result is never letting the body know what's coming next and experiencing enhanced fitness, muscle development, fat loss, and tone. Fartlek style shaking it up has the added benefit of minimizing any perceived exercise boredom.

Let's take the fartlek change principle one step further. Not only beneficial in the physical realm, "shaking it up" or "changing things up" is a great adjunct to accomplishing tone in the Fork as well as the Fun areas.

Fartlek means change is necessary for wellness development and improvement. "The only constant is change," is one of my oft repeated quotes. Repetitive, never-ending change is necessary for maximum physical, chemical, and emotional health and wellness.

Regarding nutritional chemistry (Fork), it is known that to be well fed, the types of food you fortify yourself with must be varied. This is why vegetables and fruits come in different colors, sizes, and shapes. Because they have different trace phytochemical nutritional substances. Nature wants to make them appear exciting so humans and animals take notice and graze through to internalize the varied nutritional benefits they offer. One cannot eat the same habitual routine staples and not end up deficient. Besides, that tact would be quite boring indeed.

The colorful palette of fruits and vegetables are nature's "come hither" plan to have fauna eat multitudes of different vitamins and minerals—Mother Nature's fartlek. Fartlek (oops, excuse me) is probably most beneficial in the Fun arena. The idea of boredom is most rampant in the Fun dimension and mercifully there is an easy fix, especially if like me, you have self-diagnosed ADHD tendencies. Indulge your interests. Live life like a Pinterest account. Keep a varied, energetic balance of different interests. That's why they call it Fun.

WIIFM? What's in It for Me?

High energy, restful sleep, minimized anxiety, fat loss, muscle gain, minuscule health guilt, increased flexibility, impressive endurance, enhanced strength, and, most valuable, feeling peace and contentment because you are actively progressing in the future of your own creation. The feeling of absolute certainty that you have done your best in all dimensions is difficult to describe. A deeply internalized exploding personal splendor of satisfaction comes close. I wish this for you.

The Joy of Freezing

Alert. Alert. Yet another mountain fable ahead, possibly even one with a point.

An ode swiped from my first book *Lessons From Everest: 7 Powerful Steps to the Top of Your World* illustrates personal satisfaction far from any summit.

Just shy of leaving for the summit week-long rotation on my second attempt of Mount Everest in 2008, I was freezing my fingers while doing laundry in a glacial melt-water pond near my tiny tent at Mount Everest base camp. It was a mindless busywork activity, but I needed fresh polypro socks and undertrow for the brutal hell week to come.

Suddenly out of nowhere, I experienced a deep unanticipated feeling of satisfaction. Almost like whacking your noggin on a door frame, it took a beat to figure out why. I was perfused with an intensely wonderful deep feeling of calmness, satisfaction, and awe. I was still at least a week away from any hope of achieving my goal of standing on top of the world, and the possibility of not making the top or even perishing in the attempt were distinct possibilities. Many climbers who were more skilled than myself have died on Everest over the years and their bodies remain, never to be recovered. I had no idea how my second and last attempt would work out as there existed an endless number of potential scenarios in the week ahead.

Then the powerful awakening and sudden realization of the cause of my deep content. It occurred to me, with numb fingers rubbing a bar of soap over my undies, that I had simply done everything, in the entire previous year, in the absolute best manner that I could. I had simply done my best. My fitness was awesome, my nutrition was awesome, I was in a good place mentally, but also with my family, my work, my business, my coworkers, my patients, my finances were all in the best possible shape in order for me to be there at that moment, that second, having the most warm satisfying second while my fingers were freezing.

I highly recommend the eternal search for deep feelings of satisfaction from a job well done, an intention achieved, a goal concluded, or a metaphorical mountain climbed. There is simply no match in self-satisfaction. It's not a cocky "look at me" thing, more a "from the soul" acceptance of yourself. Go ahead, reach around and give yourself a pat on the back.

Perhaps as you traverse the hills and dales of mastering Feet, Fork, and Fun you place your first tentative steps from the base camp of your present health situation to the uncertain summit of your Mount Tone, you can experience the deep satisfaction of the journey without a destination, the pursuit of which results in a happy, healthy long life.

Let's get started, shall we?

Chapter Four: Points to Ponder

1. Stress ain't necessarily bad. Accentuate the good while minimizing the bad.

2. Good stress accumulates but so does the bad. Keep alert please.

3. 3 × 3 × 3 = 6 pack. First 3 = Feet, Fork, and Fun.
   Second 3 = Increase the good aspects of the first 3.
   Third 3 = minimize the stresses of the 3 dimensions.

4. 6 pack = euphemism for tone.

5. Improving any positive stress automatically increases the vibration in all three dimensions. Minimizing even one negative stress automatically increases vibration as well.

6. Fartlek for president.

7. Self-satisfaction of following through? Priceless.

8. You want to find something? (Health) Then look for other cool stuff (energy, new relationship, a healthy weight).

Part Two "Let's Roll"

Are you guys ready? Let's Roll.—Todd Beamer 9/11/01

A Note on Change

As predictably as monarch butterflies return to Mexico, Americans stage a mass migration after January 1 to the local gym. But like the ephemeral lifespan of an insect, this dalliance with fitness is brief. By President's Day the line for the step mill is nonexistent. Why do we do this to ourselves? We do have a deep human need to self-improve but like the '70s-era Ford Pinto we seem destined to default to non-movement. A study showed 90% of heart attack victims returned to their old disease-producing lifestyle within two years. Nearly all dieters return to their former weight (or gain more) within a year.

What's up with us? Psychologists call this failing phenomenon "restraint bias." We seem to be simply overconfident with our willpower. I don't mean to say that people can't change. Some transform brilliantly and stick with it. How does one become a successful "changer"? Here's the key: successful "changers" simply accept within themselves the need to change, then act or behave like the person one wants to become. "Act as if" works. The most effective way to move toward change is to act like the healthy person who already did it. What would they do/not do? What would that winning lifestyle look like? Personally, I have noticed if I lay out my clothes and shoes for a morning walk or trip to the gym the night before it's game over... done deal. If I blow off the clothes plan, I invent wonderfully complex and logical excuses resulting in no morning workout and bruised self-esteem. No one changes their internal and external reality overnight but small incremental changes over time is what built the pyramids and carved the Grand Canyon.

CHAPTER FIVE

Feet: The Why of Moving Well

What a disgrace it is for a man to grow old without ever seeing the beauty and strength of which his body is capable.
—Socrates

> Every Week Is a Feet Week
>
> Three "hard" fitness days/week.
>
> Three "zen" fitness days/week.
>
> One rest day.
>
> Repeat every week till age 120.

Do you have 195 minutes per week to move your body? If not, how many minutes per week do you think you have before both your brain and body rot inside your skin suit? There are 168 hours in a week, which is 10,080 minutes. If you subtract 3,360 minutes, which is eight hours of sleep per night, that leaves you with 6,720 minutes of semi-discretionary time each week. Let's say your career and family demand another 4,000 minutes, lowering truly discretionary time to 2,720 minutes/week. I am here to tell you that anyone can be a personal fitness superstar of epic proportions in 195 of those minutes. This means you can be optimally fit in just 7% of your spare time. Will you? Will you find your inner superstar? And no, golf doesn't count in the minutes total if you take a cart. You're not moving well if you can smoke a cigar and suck down a beer while "exercising."

Tim's Top Ten Titillating Training Tidbits for Tone

1. Moving the body is critical for basic health and mandatory for tone. Our bodies were simply made to move and you cannot be well if you don't move well every day.

2. If you are overweight or have an active disease process, bring this book to your doctor(s) and discuss. As soon as you get the OK start moving immediately as you will live longer when active than an average-weight person who is inactive. I'll say that again. Overweight folks who exercise live longer than average weight people who don't.

Note: Non-Mountain Side Story: I ride a Trek mountain bike that is modified to protect my high mileage—induced achy parts. In years past I have participated in RAGBRAI, a 500-mile seven-day noncompetitive bike ride across the state of Iowa. The event resembles Burning Man for sixty year olds with bikes. There is a pile of fit people, obviously, but I have been amazed to observe the number of seriously overweight, even morbidly obese, cyclists riding seventy miles per day for seven days. A reminder that good hearts and arteries alone will not result in tone. A reminder that all corners of the wellness triad are necessary to be balanced, healthy, and toned.

3. Whatever level of fitness or sloth, your progress must be gradual—one step at a time to climb your Everest. Start wherever you are and whenever you are ready—for example, start right now by getting on the floor and doing a plank for as long as you can (I am). An even better idea is to start before you're ready. Just go. Don't underdo life by overthinking life. Be "wickit smaht" as they say in Rhode Island, and if you are in the beginning stages of a fitness plan and an activity doesn't feel right, swap it out with a similar activity. Never force anything. There are unlimited possibilities of potential activities (Google "functional training"). If one exercise activity doesn't float your boat, don't skip the workout, adapt instead.

4. Do you poo poo walking? Too wimpy for you perhaps? Try these two walks on for size. The first one is the Dr. Tim Walkabout (capitalized because it is way more than a zen walk). Start with a mini Walk-about in the morning or evening or both and include family and/or friends. The point of the world famous Walkabout is to get outside, vary the terrain, vary the speed, breathe deep, get out of breath, catch your breath, repeatedly climb hills, sing a song, wave and smile to everybody, pet all the friendly dogs, run here and there if you wish, observe what has changed since your last stroll (there is always something different), wear a pack with weight in it sometimes, watch the plants grow or the leaves fall off, bounce a tennis ball on

pavement sometimes then catch it while you walk, do some carioca, side shuffles, and other fun activities from my QuickFit routine, jump over a log, drop and plank (see my website for videos of me performing a smattering of the various activities at www.drtimwarren.com) for thirty seconds at three telephone poles in a row, do some bear crawling. Make up your own cool stuff to do and change it every time out the door. Fartlek the whole thing. Practice smiling and cultivate contentment. Just be! Side Note: I live a mile off a sleepy country road in Rhode Island and on my Walkabouts I noticed that hardly anybody waved in greeting. I then decided to wave at every oncoming car including landscapers, school buses, and FedEx drivers regardless of the response. In short order everybody waved back. People stuck in their habits just needed an excuse. I changed the culture single handedly. You can, too. Go as long and as far as you can. Under a time constraint? Set your phone alarm for half the time you have then turn around and beat your time on the way home.

The second is called a Dr. Tim Zen Walk. (Have you noticed how incredibly famous I am? Not one but two walks named after yours truly.) In this one there is no fitness agenda as it's more of a mental cleansing. A gentle stroll on the beach, on grass, in your garden, or in the city. Revel in gentle movement outdoors. It's preferred to minimize hard surfaces, in fact, go barefoot as much as possible. Grass playing fields at high schools and colleges work well but your back yard is acceptable. Be safe and revel in dirty feet. If you must wear athletic shoes make sure you buy ones that you try on and they feel simply awesome, in the store, while wearing the style sock you will exercise in. Never buy an athletic shoe because you dig the funky color. If you are indeed starting from scratch with activity level, work your way up in distance slowly, but vary the speed and hilliness if possible. All steps are a waystation to your summit.

"Damn, it's raining" you say? Newsflash. There is a new invention called the raincoat.

It is not because things are difficult that we do not dare, it is because we do not dare that they are difficult.—Seneca

5. There is planned (scheduled like an important appointment) exercise and unplanned exercise, or a combination. Learn what works best for your lifestyle and your headspace, but develop the openness to utilize both for best results. It's helpful to plan or even semi-plan your day especially if you are the most disorganized person on earth. If you are the most organized person on earth then maybe you need to ease up a little, exercise your improvisational muscles and cultivate your "feel" for daily workouts. In my experience, doing some fitness activities first thing in the morning has the big benefits of being performed before inevitable emergencies or distractions rob minutes later on in the day. Feeling good? Push it. Feeling iihh? Back it off or change it around. Additionally, it is a very fine feeling indeed to know your exercise is done, or even mostly done. You are one up on the world when you move your bod first thing. Mornings are great for calorie burning, but, again, best of all is the fun, fun, fun that comes from having climbed your Everest right away, leaving the rest of your day for further adventures. Lots of folks who are overly rigid miss a scheduled sweat session then don't make it up. Shoot for three main quality ("hard") workouts/week that way you can still see great results without the feeling of giving up.

6. If you have kids or grandkids, you know the benefit of facilitating play as often as possible and off the devices. If you are older, I believe that you need to regress to childhood and start playing again. Preferably outside. We do not grow old and stop playing—we stop playing then grow old. The Walkabout is play but it can also be one of your three "hard"/week. My "Homer" and "TV 20" workouts are play, hell all my stuff is play. The "Homer" is a series of exercises using a five-gallon bucket from Home Depot and the "TV 20" is a workout that can be done during the twenty minutes of commercials typical in an hour of TV.

7. Athletic Position.

   Do you do yard work, housework, play second base for the Red Sox, or coach under-six soccer? Do you want to have rock hard abdominal muscles without doing one sit up? Then know and love the Athletic Position.

- Look forward.
- Close your mouth.
- Touch your tongue to the roof of your mouth.
- Chin back.
- Keep your head and spine gently aligned.
- Tighten up your abs, as if someone was going to punch you in the stomach.
- Knees bent slightly.
- Feet shoulder-width apart.
- Keep the weight of your shoulders and your elbows down.
- Relax body and mind.

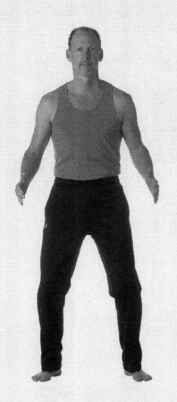
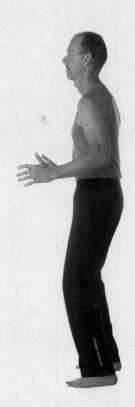

Stay aware of this athletic, ready-for-anything, default position before, during, and after vacuuming your pad or Sunday's playing defensive end. This position helps you feel serious about what you are doing, which is developing your inner and outer athlete. It is stabilizing for injury prevention, it facilitates performance, it stimulates focus on fitness, and supports a new improved body awareness. It makes a mountain out of you and if you keep at it, it will result in rock hard abs even if there is a layer of jiggly adipose tissue on top of those beauties. Side note: while walking, tighten your abs and walk for a telephone pole length. Rest a length then do it again. Keep adding telephone poles then carry the telephone pole. OK, just joshing on that last one.

Getting stronger makes you weightless.—The Author

8. The U.S. Centers for Disease Control and Prevention (CDC) found only 20% of Americans got their recommended exercise amount: 150 minutes of moderate intensity aerobic activity or 75 minutes of vigorous intensity activity per week plus strength training twice/week. In total minutes this is roughly the same total as my 195 minutes/week plan but my intention is to have you do both moderate and vigorous and not either/or in addition to the twice weekly strength. How can you tell if activity is moderate or vigorous? Heart rate.

   You can measure your heart rate with any of the myriad heart rate monitors available or stop and count your carotid pulse or go by how you breathe. A rough way to compare moderate vs vigorous is that with vigorous you are out of breath while having an actual or virtual conversation. Having a conversation with a real or imaginary friend during moderate activity means not being particularly out of breath. Simple. If you resist wearable exercise gizmos, do a combo of attention to breath and pulse taking.

9. Visualize your successful fitness. Don't forget that a great many people have accomplished what you desire and many have failed. Does someone who you admire pop into mind? It doesn't matter if it's, "Wow, I really admire that person's physique or accomplishment," or, "If that assbucket can accomplish that then I certainly can."

Inspiration is inspiration so don't question, just do. Many clients use a motivating picture on their intention card. Use this powerful mind-body connection technique. Your essence can't tell the difference between reality and what is vividly imagined so intend the results you wish. You can achieve whatever you intend but once again don't overthink. Truth be told I can overthink a cup of coffee, so I'm telling myself while brow-beating you.

Intend to exercize more for performance rather than aesthetics as they are more rewarding and less ephemeral. Examples: driving a golf ball farther, lifting heavier, beating a 5K time, entering and completing an obstacle race. Aesthetics take care of themselves with a toned lifestyle anyway.

Warning: You Knew It Was Coming

On my first Everest climb, I could not visualize myself on the summit due to fear and doubt. Because of this fear and doubt combined with the mind-body connection, I became quite ill with a lung and throat infection. Possibly, my illness gave me an "out" so I wouldn't have to face my fear of surviving Everest. I had observed this phenomenon with mountaineers on other great peaks around the world. I made the intelligent but distressing call of quitting the climb that year but a remarkable thing happened. A guy who I didn't expect at all to get close, not only got to the top but safely down. Until that particular teammate succeeded I could not see myself at the top. Once I observed this particular friend succeed and thought about it for a few days, I was all aboard mentally for the next year's climbing attempt and was ultimately successful. I don't know how or why this particular bro became my motivation but who cares? If he could do it then I could too. The lesson here is to find someone to model that resonates with your soul and keep putting one foot in front of the other in your Everest climb of life.

Shake it till the butter melts, shake it till the butter melts, shake that cosmic thing, shake that thing, shake it, oh yea.
—The B-52's

Do you have mentor in mind? A picture or two will really help. Find a picture of someone who really inspires you in some way. It could be someone you know or it could be a picture from a magazine or somewhere. Post it as your screen shot on your cell, desktop, refrigerator, and on your journal that arrives with your Everest 70 Challenge kit.

Post it everywhere so that you won't waver on your goal. Imaginary mentors work too, mix and match attributes if you wish.

10. No pain, no gain.

No pain, no gain? How about yes and no? There are varying amounts of discomfort in the process of getting fit—even strong discomfort. I recall being on a long hot bike ride with a buddy years ago and I was silently bumming out about the "pain" I was experiencing as I ascended a long gradual hill. I was really convincing myself of my victimhood. Then it occurred to me that it wasn't pain at all, rather it was "discomfort." I would persevere. I would survive. Almost immediately the pain was gone and the discomfort was barely noticeable. I flew over the remaining hills and dales and never forgot this lesson. Ask yourself about the discomfort/pain conundrum the next time you want to quit in any endeavor, the "pain" may be psychic and not physical at all. If you determine that "pain" in fact exists, change what you are doing or stop and reassess. Actual discomfort is fine, even welcomed, actual pain may not be. Pain could be damage to joints, muscles, or bone.

Change is hardest at the beginning, messiest in the middle, and best at the end.—Robin Sharma

I love a little DOMS—delayed onset muscle soreness—with my coffee. DOMS is that minor muscle soreness one or two days after a workout. I like DOMS as it lets me know I am accomplishing something. However, there is no purpose to immobilizing muscle pain found in really overdoing it. That's damage. I've made this mistake occasionally and it ain't pretty. Discomfort during or after exercise = Gain = you are winning. Pain during or after exercise = Damage = you are a big dope. You are the only one who can accurately gauge if you are a winner or a big dope. When in doubt, ask the gorgeous athlete in the mirror. There are a few things that can help decrease the severity of DOMS: calcium and magnesium supplements, warming up properly, hydration before and during activity, post session stretching, and drinking a post session protein drink containing the amino acid glutamine within two hours.

Fitness Data Dump

If more information was the answer, then we'd all be billionaires with perfect abs.—Derek Sivers

The intent of this book is not to be the end-all be-all compilation of contemporary fitness, nutrition, and headspace research and information available today. No one could dead lift such a book. I would have to sell a sturdy piece of oaken furniture to display and turn the pages of the hypothetical mighty tome. (Wait a minute, that's an excellent idea.) I am supplying physical, chemical, and philosophical tenets that worked for me and 10,000 other folks in my office and, though based on science, I suggest you study for the rest of your days to increase knowledge about exercise and nutrition and headspace (feet, fork, and fun). Incorporate what makes sense and eliminate what does not. Science, technology, and understanding will always develop over time but principles, ethics, and universal truths are timeless. Keep learning till you die then enjoy that next adventure.

Gradually progress through ebbs and flows of motivation, time constraints, and other hiccups, and remember that health takes lifelong attention and never involves the fallacy of seeking perfection.

Have you noticed that some people like strawberry ice cream and some like chocolate? Have you noticed that some people have different body shapes than others? Factor in that people have unique genetic potentials. Then how would it be possible for there to be a one-size-fits-all exercise routine? We must listen to our bodies and pay constant attention to the discomfort/pain balance.

All my exercise life there have been certain activities that my body hated. Activities that felt horrible to my knees, lower back, shoulders, or spine. I didn't question it; I just stayed away. For example, dead lifts for my glutes, back, and legs or military presses for my shoulders are verboten in my world. They feel like my bones and joints will pop out of my skin and fly across the room like sticking a pin into a balloon. However, dead lifts for Sally or Steve could be completely awesome and they hate lunges or ab rolls. Your body will tell you. I urge you to practice doing the same. There are hundreds and thousands of ways to properly move body parts in an exercise fashion so don't worry if one or two hate you. Become adept at listening to your body without interjecting laziness or sloth into the equation. At my present age of fifty-six there are an increasing number of activities that are now on my no-go list. However, I have added dozens of fun, new, albeit easier, activities to the ever changing mix. I do my best to balance a stimulating training response while at the same time listening to the messages from various parts of my body that scream the loudest—no forcing and no hating.

Gentlemen... Start Your Lawnmowers

In activities of daily living (ADLs) like taking out the trash, pulling the towels from the washing machine, yelling and screaming at a T-ball game from the stands, or starting your lawnmower the body moves in multiple planes. Therefore, the focus of exercise in the Feet dimension should be in multiple planes, otherwise called functional training. Wikipedia has a slightly more general definition, "Functional Training (or Functional Fitness) is a classification of exercise which involves training the body for the activities performed in daily life."

Let's Talk About the Gym, Tim

Going to the local muscle head gym to develop individual muscles for endless hours may be your thing but wellness is something different. Also, traditional bodybuilding exercises don't translate to starting your lawnmower. I used to laugh in my fraternity days at the hard core bodybuilders in the house who would not carry the beer kegs into the house as it would "ruin" their training. It was left to the skinny, non-anal-retentive brothers of Pi Kappa Chi to wrestle the 160-pound libation cans for the next Duke Kahanamoku bash.

Functional training is exercise that involves training the body for activities performed in daily life. This involves weight bearing and off balance activities, targeting core muscles of the abdomen, lower back and the glutes, manipulating awkward objects, etc. Balance activities are often utilized as well to train the primary system for life—the brain and nervous system. Again, I refer you to www.drtimwarren.com for videos of my favorite balance and functional activities.

My gym is Planet Fitness. I love the everybody welcome mindset and I crack up over the "lunk alarm" inside. I also love the $10/month dues. With that said, its purpose is not functional training. I love the Step Mill (the tall machine with the movable steps) lots. Superb moderate exercise but very easily blown into the vigorous mode (and I can fantasize of climbing another 8,000-meter Himalayan peak). I like the strength machines also (I know, I know, I just touted the benefits of functional). Once/week, more or less, I blow into the Planet and run through either an upper or lower machine circuit. Change and variety is Fartlek folks, a fun part of Feet.

Despite the fact I previously disparaged the bodybuilding as being nonfunctional, everybody should construct and maintain muscle. This book will give instruction in the care, feeding, and maintenance of muscle from adulthood to the last known adventure of life: the Cubs winning the World Series. Speaking of the end of all days...

I See Dead People (with embarrassing muscle tone)

Please help stamp out and eliminate redundancy (as well as sarcopenia). Sarcopenia is the loss of muscle size and strength due to aging and being a couch yam. Couch yam syndrome is a name I just made up for the unfortunate and embarrassing default condition for too many. Sarcopenia is so average, boring, and dangerous that it must be stopped. How do we stop sarcopenia? Moving well, Eating well, Thinking well, and Sleeping well. All will be revealed, stay tuned.

As a student at Palmer College of Chiropractic in the early 1980s, my favorite classes involved dissection lab. Finally, after years of undergraduate and graduate book work, I could study real human structure. The cadavers in those days were harder to study than today's advances in the body preparation for professionals in the healing arts. Nowadays there are synthetic cadavers for study, great computer programs, even the incredibly beautiful specimens in those BodyWorld traveling exhibits.

So anyway, I am a twenty-four-year-old kid in a white lab coat in anatomy lab carrying a little box with scalpels and probes. The barren, unadorned antiseptic room holds a dozen stainless steel tanks with a human body in each one that lab assistants would crank up to drain the fluids out. The first one was a sixty-something-year-old lady who must have weighed eighty pounds. Once myself and my fellow chiropractors in training teased the quadriceps muscle out from skin, fascia, and connective tissue this lady's main muscle in the front of the upper leg was no bigger in circumference than an average sized thumb.

Sarcopenia. Caused by a lifetime of poor health choices namely inactivity and poor nutrition. This lady's muscles looked like she would barely have had the power to sit up, and I was correct of course because she was dead as a doornail. The next cadaver was a twenty-something African-American man who died in an accident. After prepping his quads they popped out like steel bars. You could easily discern the striations of the four distinct muscle bellies that make up the quadriceps group. He must have been using those muscles heartily, had better nutrition, and, to be fair, he was younger. What knocked me over with a feather was not the smell but the third body. An eighty-something-year-old lady, tiny in stature but really nice quads (I was going to suggest "nice legs" but that would have been weird—surely I would have received disapproving stares by my student brothers and sisters). This lady's wheels were smaller than the young man's but not by that much! Lesson learned: aging is optional. Yes. I know she was also dead but I am hypothesizing she had a more active and fun life than the sixty-something lady with sarcopenia.

The process of sarcopenia is not inevitable as we march down the trail of getting older. If you minimize sitting, move your body regularly including at least two short muscle-strengthening sessions, and follow Chapter Seven, Fork, to nutritionally support your physiology you significantly decrease the muscle-withering process of sarcopenia.

Did your mother admonish you to change your underwear because you might end up in the hospital? She may have been less concerned with you in the hospital than implying your dirty u-trow would reflect badly on her parenting prowess. The motherly admonition should be "Think, Train, Eat, and Sleep properly so you don't have a gaggle of grad students with judgmental expressions snickering at your embarrassing sarcopenia in dissection lab."

Big Picture Alert

Have you been overwhelmed with trying to start or maintain an exercise program? Have you had trouble finding the time to move? Have you been angry at yourself or depressed or anxiety ridden as a result? Have I added to your unease? Strength training, walking, walkabouts, cardiovascular work, flexibility, HIIT, Zumba, Yoga, sprinting, Cross-Fit, blah, blah blah. There is so much data and recommendations out there in the exercise, diet, and headspace arena that people are often confused, anxiety ridden, depressed, or all three. Take your foot off the gas, put your mind in neutral, and apply some metaphoric pressure to the brake pedal for a moment and realize that we all will gravitate to different interests and actions throughout our adventure here on earth. It's all cool. Just do something today and something a little different tomorrow.

With the above statement made, folks should do as many different and varied activities as possible because that aligns with our hunter-gatherer DNA and essence. Besides, it keeps us from getting bored and being boring. The great thing about functional training is you get the big ticket components of cardio, strength, flexibility, and balance all at the same time and if you add a couple of wilderness or urban hikes, bike rides, Dr. Tim walkabouts, ball room dances, or yoga sessions per week then you win. You are climbing the health continuum to your lofty mountain summit.

Chapter Five: Brain Train Exercise

Why You Are a Miracle, In Case You Forgot

Improbability that humans are "mistakes."

(This is deep, so bear with me.)

Age of the universe: 10 to the tenth power years old or 10 to the eighteenth power seconds old.

Specificity of hemoglobin (part of a blood cell): 10 to the six hundred fiftieth power.

Specificity of DNA in T4 cell (a smaller part of a cell): 10 to the seventy-eighth power.

David Foster, *The Philosophical Scientists* (1993)

What does the above mean to you?

Chapter Five: Points to Ponder

1. One hundred and ninety-five minutes (195) out of ten thousand and eighty (10,080).
2. Know and love athletic position. Tighten your tummy throughout your day.
3. Love, care, and grow your muscles till age 120.
4. Move functionally.

CHAPTER SIX

Feet: The How of Moving Well

Everything you do is more than none. —The Author

Feet Week Options

Hard Days (3/week)	Zen Days (2-3/week)	Rest Days (1-2/week)
Sprints: 1-2×/week	QuickFit routine	Zen walks
LSD: 1×/week	Planes/balance	Planes/balance
Trad weight training	Golf: walking	Golf: cart
AMRAP 1-2×/week	Yoga/Tai Chi	Brain wake-up routines
TV20: 1-3×/week	Rock climbing gym	Housework
Class: CrossFit, Zumba, etc	Dr. Tim Walkabout	Gardening

Muscle 101

There are endless ways you can perform strength, cardio, and flexibility work. I recommend a mix and match style to keep the body guessing and not to get into a rut physiologically or mentally. We are in the fitness game for the rest of our life and health, as we have learned, is a dynamic continuum. My big hairy point is we all need constant variety and change. Let's all say the "F" word together now... F******.

My second favorite word is kaizen. Kaizen is the Japanese principle for constant and never ending improvement. I believe it originated in the Japanese business world when they turned "Made In Japan" from a joke to gold in less than a generation. Incidentally, it was an American, Edward Deming, who was a consultant to the country post-WWII who was instrumental in the progression.

Change, variety, and the resulting personal growth are all axioms of kaizen. In the arena of fitness training, my interpretation of kaizen correlates with not ever getting stuck in the same routine for more than two weeks... tops! When I was training for my second and ultimately successful Mount Everest climb I worked a plan with my trainer to never do the same workout sequence ever—for one whole year. Each day was entirely different. The plan was to never let my body know what was coming next in order to be as resilient, powerful, and ready for anything as possible. That sounds good to you in the wilds of suburbia, doesn't it? Constant never ending improvement of body, chemistry, and mind. The precept of kaizen is useful as affirmation so feel free to incorporate it into your self-talk, intentions, and belief system.

Heaven moves steadily. So should man exercise himself regularly.
—The I-Ching

Base Camp to Summit

While wearing a silver smoking jacket and sipping Cabernet, I've spent many an evening deep in thought. First, there are endless exercise combinations and variations; second, there are endless and varied types of human beings; and, third, these humans exhibit endless and varied experience and fitness levels. How the heck do I share a simple, step-by-step workout plan without making my audience slam the book shut and throw it at their cat? Easy. Apparently most of my readers are dog people.

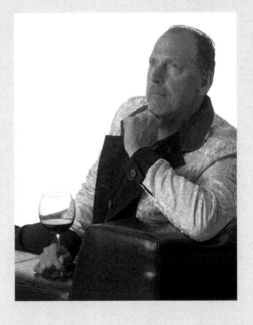

There are multiple levels of fitness and activity within Feet but they are not carved in stone and blend into each other as fitness progresses. There is no benefit getting hung up on what level you are in at the moment. In fact, a superstar professional athlete can get benefit from the Base Camp QuickFit Base Camp series even if it is just for an innovative warm up. All levels involve some cardio (activity that raises heart and respiration rate), strength (muscles contract as maximally as possible), and flexibility (activity that supports tendon, ligament, and joint limberness). The cool thing is that many functional training activities include cardio, strength, and flexibility simultaneously. Fitness one-stop shopping. Let's get to it, shall we?

The Week in Feet

3 Hard Days. 3 Zen Days. 1 Rest Day. = 7 Days/Week Till 120.

That's the plan in a nutshell. I could attempt to BS you and say you could get by with less but this 195 minute/week schedule is required to reverse dis-ease trends and climb the mountain of tone.

FAQ #1: "What makes a hard day?"

A: Hard days and zen days are alternated and are determined by your heart rate. Your heart rate is determined by one of the many personal heart rate monitors available or, for free, by your pointer and middle fingers checking the neck (carotid) or wrist (radial) pulses. Stop exercise and count the pulses for 30 or 60 seconds. If 30 multiply by two to get your heart rate.

FAQ #2: "What should my pulse be on hard or zen days?"

A: For "zen" or moderate-intensity days, a person's heart rate (HR) should be 50% to 70% of his or her maximum HR. The maximum HR is based on age. The common estimate formula for max HR is 220—age [50 years] = 170 heart beats/minute (BPM). Therefore, the 50% and 70% levels would be: $170 \times 0.50 = 85$ BPM and $170 \times 0.70 = 119$ BPM, respectively. Thus, for a 50-year-old shooting for a Zen moderate-intensity day, the target HR should be between 85 and 119 during the workout.

For hard days or vigorous-intensity days, a target HR should be between 70% and 85% of max HR. Following the above calculations but using the different percentages, a thirty-five-year-old would have a max HR of 220 - 35 = 185 BPM and the 70% and 85% levels would be: $185 \times 0.70 = 130$ BPM and: $185 \times 0.85 = 157$ BPM, respectively. Therefore, a thirty-five-year-old will have a target HR of between 130 and 157.

FAQ #3: "What if I can't even spell math and I don't want a heart rate gizmo?"

A: Go with the breath/conversation determination. If you can carry on a conversation without getting winded, chances are you are in zen day training. If you are winded while speaking with your imaginary friend during exercise, congrats, you are a nutcase performing vigorous or hard day training.

FAQ #4: "Dr. Tim, your 195 minutes/week hard/zen plan differs a bit from the CDC recommendations, doesn't it?"

A: Yep. In my opinion we athletes of tone need more time spent moving than the CDC suggests.

FAQ #5: "How long should I exercise per workout?"

A: Again, discuss with your health care professional if you are just beginning any fitness program but I would start with 10-15 minutes for hard workout days (after warming up) and 20-40 minutes for zen days. For the more experienced fitness devotee, head toward 40 minutes for hard days and 40-60 for zen days.

Feet: The Long View

Some folks will primarily bike, some will run, some will swim (Tri-heads will do all three), some will Zumba, some will pump the iron, some will CrossFit, some will hike, and some will fight bulls. Since it's not my mission to share all the fitness knowledge ever dreamed up, I suggest a starting program that requires only basic equipment rescued from the nooks and crannies of the average garage or basement and many fitness activities don't even require that.

In a Feet Week workout, clients accomplish cardio, strength, flexibility, brain training, and myofascial release. I will use the series of camps on a Mount Everest climb as analogy of a particular exercise's exertion level. Let's begin.

Dr. Tim's Base Came to Camp 4 Fitness Definitions

Base Camp at 17,300 feet on Mount Everest's south side in Nepal is a place for recuperation for the mountaineer between bouts of heavy exertion while climbing at the above Camps 1 to 4 on the way to the summit at 29,035 feet. Using the analogy of the progressively harder (physically and mentally) camps as harder exercise days, I have mentioned and recommend a typical week of three hard days (exertion and intensity roughly like camps 3-4) followed by two to three easy (zen days) days/week of a lessened intensity such as camps 1-2 in intensity or duration then one to two days at base camp (rest days). There is an infinite number of activities, exercises, and workouts just like there is an endless number of differences in people attempting to work out. I will not attempt to write a fitness encyclopedia here but rather my take on the big picture then the student of tone can use some creativity and their own personal preferences in designing the work out plan. Many of my fave exercises are demonstrated on video at www.drtimwarren.com.

AMRAP (as many reps as possible): Concept of doing an activity until you can't do one more repetition using proper form. (Also known as "failure"—a concept I am so fond of I put it in the subtitle.)

Balance: Brain and nervous system exercise by encouraging instability. Usually standing.

Camps 1-4: Progression of exercise difficulty as defined by you, the climber of tone. Too hard? Back off a tad. Too easy? Add time, repetitions, weight, or decrease rest time.

Cardio: Activity that gets the heart and breathing rate elevated. Examples: swimming, biking, or running.

Core: Group of activities targeting the front and sides of the abdomen as well as back muscles and hips.

Fartlek: switching up intensity, usually in cardio. For example, one could be enjoying an LSD day then by throwing in a sprint series, it becomes a fartlek (I wanted to use the word twice).

Hard/Zen: A harder exercise day is followed with easier rest day activities. In my average week fitness recommendations, I advocate for three hard days, two to three zen days, and one to two rest days. There is always a zen day or rest day or even two following a hard day.

Homers: Exercises done using a five-gallon Home Depot bucket.

LSD: Long slow distance. A cardio and zen day where the distance is increased but the intensity is low. It can be a hard day if you go 25% longer than usual as an example.

Planes: Activities involving moving the spine in all directions: forward, backward, side to side, and most importantly (completely lacking in many folks' routines) rotationally.

QuickFit Base Camp: Warm-up routine for established "climbers" or hard day exercises for beginners.

Sprints: 30-20-10 × 5. Once warmed up a series of five cardio repetitions of 30 seconds at 50% effort, then 20 seconds at 75%, followed by 10 seconds at 90%+ effort done five complete times on your choice of cardio activity.

Trad: Common free weight or machine body building exercises.

TV 20: Grouping of exercises that can be done in the twenty minutes of commercials in the typical hour of TV.

Important note: There are infinite combinations of fantastic fitness activities available and it is not the purpose of this book to be a compendium of all. Once again, see a sample workout week on my website at www.drtimwarren.com.

The QuickFit Base Camp Routine

Again with the Mountain Analogy: Base Camp on the Nepal side of Mount Everest sits at 17,500 feet on a fractured, constantly moving thick sheet of Khumbu Glacier ice within a cirque of the Himalayan giants Pumori, Nuptse, and the West Shoulder of Everest. An ephemeral hovel of a hundred or so tents serves as the hub and home of the aspiring summiteer. It's where climbers spend the bulk of the seventy days necessary to acclimatize and lick the physical and psychic wounds of attempting mountaineering's holy grail. Base Camp is the beginning of your metaphoric Everest climb up the wellness continuum. These dozen and a half moves are both introductory and advanced as they are a workout to aspire to for beginners or athletes who have been away from physical activity for a while, as well as a complete program for the intro and intermediate athlete, and a solid warm-up for the superstar demographic. Although you can add and subtract many activities in Base Camp, its basic structure serves as a go-to work out when in doubt.

Thanks to Matt Hopkins, DPT, and wife/trainer Becky, proprietors of Hop's Athletic Performance, for years of instruction, inspiration, and perspiration in the performance of many of the following activities (and for looking out for my troublesome back). See them demonstrated at www.drtimwarren.com.

1. Perform my "two-minute brain wake-up call" exercises as a warm-up to the warm-up and to remind you they exist and should be done as often as possible (preferably once/hour of sitting).

2. Walking knee hugs.

3. Walking glute stretches.

4. Walking calf raises.

5. Walking hip circles.

6. Side shuffles each side.

7. Shuffle with leg crossing over in front both sides and

8. Shuffle sides with leg crossing midline in rear.

9. Carioca.

10. Walking quad stretch.

11. Walking high kick. (These first 11 activities are done out and back, assuming a thirty-foot exercise area).

12. Thirty-second jumping jacks.

13. Thirty-second seal jumping jacks.

14. Thirty-second split jumps.

15. Thirty second plyometric jump in place.

16. Ten pushups.

17. Ten squats.

18. Ten lunges on each leg.

19. Check your pulse and finish with.

20. P-Knot and/or foam roll session (more about myofascial release in Chapter Ten, The Everest 70 Challenge).

For regular exercisers, the Base Camp series is a great warm-up for a Camps 2, 3, or 4 training session; for folks just beginning a fitness program or have been away from it for a while, it may be too hard to complete Base Camp right away. It doesn't matter. Just do what you can do using your discomfort vs. pain internal guide. Remember that? If you can't do regular pushups, for example, then do them on your knees. Need to be shown? Don't understand the exercise? Want to make absolutely sure you are doing them properly? Consider my Everest 70 Challenge coaching option where I work one on one with people online or my EverWrest two-day coaching program in person. See descriptions of both at my website.

Did you notice something different about the Base Camp routine? It may be that it's a functional routine although you may not have affixed that label. Did you feel some stretching? Did you feel muscular exertion? Was it hard to keep your balance at times? All of the above? You accomplished brain stimulation, strength, flexibility, and cardio just in the Base Camp routine. Reach around and pat yourself on the back for even more flexibility. Greasing the joints; de-greasing the circulation; building hard muscle; blasting jiggly fat; developing flexibility; minimizing physical, chemical, and emotional negative stress; maximizing physical, chemical, and emotional positive stress; and brain training exercise? You are a multitasking Feet, Fork, and Fun fanatic.

Own your fitness. Anyone can be tough. The greatest gift you can give yourself is to train every day and seek new challenges. The effort you put forth is all on you.—Rorke Denver, Navy SEAL commander

Over the decades I have experienced and researched an endless number of endurance and strength training programs involving gaggles of gadgets and gizmos but by far my favorite is to use your own body weight with minimal equipment. You can do this too. I could stroll into your garage or basement and, besides decent footwear, have all the free exercise equipment we would ever need. When body weight exercise techniques are used and overcoming gravitational pull is harnessed, the minimalist cave-person athlete can garner stupendous gains in strength, cardio, and flexibility. Additionally, it's free. No doodad costs or gym fees unless you have proven to yourself that you are serious about your personal health revolution. As a matter of fact, I highly recommend that you don't spend one penny, including on my Everest 70 Challenge, not one cent, unless and until you prove to yourself that you are serious about lifestyle improvement. This takes successful health focus of over three weeks' duration.

Warm It Up

The purpose of a warm-up is to ease into increased circulation, cajole the heart and respiration rates higher, and to initiate some glow (perspiration). Apparently, the process of sweating has hired a poor public relations firm resulting in the age-old idea that our bodies leaking fluid as a result of exercise is something to be avoided. Sweating profusely while being knighted by the Queen or when I am presented the Medal of Freedom wouldn't be fun, but leaking from your pores should be celebrated in most other cases. However, don't confuse sweating with the quality of a workout. After all, some people drip just thinking about exercise. I love to sweat in workouts any time of the year as I visualize sweating as a bath from the inside out. Out you damn toxins!

It takes me roughly ten minutes on the step mill at Planet Fitness or the ten minutes it takes to complete the QuickFit Base Camp routine before I get moist. Once again the routine is a balanced workout for home or yard with required space of thirty × ten feet, preferably where the chances are slim of tripping over anything. At a gym use a piece of cardio equipment that involves both upper and lower body motion such as a bike that has arm motion or a rowing machine.

Don't ask for time for yourself. If you ask, people can say no. If you just do it, then you've done it and you've got it. Your being happy is the only change they'll notice.—Dr. Mira Kirshenbaum

Caveman DNA

Right about now we have to get something straight. We have to have a little talk. It's an important topic that looms large for this chapter and the next. First, DNA (deoxyribonucleic acid) is the building block of life on earth. Our DNA makes us human. A carp's DNA makes it swim around and be a carp. Crabgrass in my garden has the DNA of crabgrass.

DNA does evolve and change over millennia but our human DNA hasn't changed a lick in at least 50,000 years. So if our DNA, or our human-ness, hasn't changed much in tens of thousands of years, has our lifestyle in the form of activity and diet changed? Should you ask the great anthropologist Michael J. Fox in *Back to the Future*? Of course human activity and nutrition and lifestyle have changed incredibly over the millennia. Lifestyle has been crazy different in the last fifty years let alone 50,000. Here's the rub. We inhabit the same meat suit hanging on a stardust frame zipping through time and space as our caveman ancestors did but we live our lives fundamentally different than our DNA essence. The result of living a life-style not in harmony with our DNA is not pretty. Refer again to the death, inflammation, and diseased mayhem that is our present culture (as discussed in Chapter Three, Have a Nice Decay). To make it worse the disease trends are worsening. The answer, then, is to eat a diet and move a body as close to the way Beverly and Bob Caveman did.

Bob: "Beverly! What's for dinner, I'm starving?" Beverly: "Same as every day Bob, chutes, roots, and ribs." Bob: "My fave! How was your day Bev?" Beverly: "Well I put little Betina Caveman on my head, walked five miles to gather firewood, then picked a pile of fruit and beat up a sabre tooth tiger. How about you Bob?" Bob: "Well, I napped under a tree until a deer-looking animal walked by then I threw rocks and sticks at it, sprinted after it on and off for hours till the beast fell over, then I carried it home." Beverly Caveman: "You are a lazy bum."

The point I wish to make is that movements illustrated by the caveman family including core strength, cardio, strength, balance, sprinting, and flexibility—all done daily by our Paleolithic ancestors— are more needed than ever in today's world. We don't have to manhandle an antelope but we sure need to fight off disease and physical entropy. Congruency must exist between exercise choices and our ancient DNA ancestry in order to achieve and maintain tone. Note: you will learn in Chapter Seven, Fork, that the same philosophy is true in nutrition.

Running Wild

Old Guy Reminiscing Alert: I started running in 1972 at the age of twelve and stopped at age forty-four when I looked around and noticed I had a shaggy beard, worn-out Nikes and a gaggle of people following me. No wait, that was Tom Hanks. As a runner, starting at age twelve, and running competitively all the way through junior high, high school, college, post-college, and until I was in my early forties, running was the major part of my fitness life. In my early years, I thought I was really in shape. As a teen I could run a twenty-six-mile marathon faster than most trained adults. My resting pulse occasionally dipped to the low-40s. I was badass, or so I thought.

As I have learned since, although I was a boss in cardiovascular health, I was not toned. I was not super fit. I had minimal core strength, I had little upper body strength, my flexibility was poor, my nutrition was cheap beer. And, I was using just two planes of movement. My spine and nervous system, intimately connected, were rigid, interfered with, and unwell.

I added swimming, biking, and traditional weight training to the mix as I moved on to triathlon competitions. I believed using the different muscle groups rather than the same ones all the time with running would be all the change needed. Better. I was moving up the tone mountain but I was leaving out some critical steps. Unwittingly, I was failing at fitness.

In my professional life, I was always a "seminar junkie." I loved learning the latest science, research, and philosophy of things natural. However, it was not until I attended a conference given by Dr. James Chestnut in the early 2000s that I saw the errors of my ways in my personal fitness and, as a result, became a much better doctor. What I learned was the importance of firing or stimulating what are called "mechanoreceptors" to stimulate the brain. With a start I realized that in my first four decades of what I thought was awesome fitness, I was, in reality, kind of a weenie. Sitting in that class I committed to the change necessary to be balanced and truly fit and to share the pathway to as many people as possible. I will not allow you, my student of tone, to make the same mistakes.

Fly Your Planes

The missing aspect to my training was a biggie. I was missing maximum brain and nervous system stimulation. This despite having seen a chiropractor between one and four times a month since I was a teen and experienced the resultant brain and nervous system power. I was missing self-induced brain and nervous system fitness because I was missing the entire plane of motion of rotation (gentle twisting motion of the spine from neck to lower back). All my iron pumping, running, biking, and, to a lesser extent, swimming were in the same old same old planes of motion. None involved rotation. Rotation is the primary plane of motion to initiate a kind of "pump" of nutrients and stimulation to the brain. I was reed thin, 10% body fat, six-pack abs, sub-three-hour marathoner, bench presser of 100 pounds more than my body weight, and I was failing at fitness. My brain, my computer, my most important organ and system which gets up to 90% of its nutrient pump from movement of the spine, was not toned. But it soon would be. Yours will be, too, if you rotate the spine daily and get checked regularly by a chiropractor.

The Greatest Exercises of All Time

If you had no time for any other fitness, I would perform either tai chi or yoga because they are one-stop shopping—movement in all planes, full body, strength, and (minimally) cardio. There is an added bonus of a meditative zen-ish calming resulting in a tight package of physical and mental fitness in a minimal period of time. A Walkabout with multiple functional activities thrown in such as "Heismans" and "The Bad Wedding Dance" thrown in would also be an impressive balanced package with more emphasis on cardio but with a brain stimulating mindfulness component.

Every movement is valuable—yard work, gardening, splitting firewood, playing tag with a pile of screaming kids. Especially a pile of kids. I once prepared for a successful ascent of Mount Rainier simply by road biking and playing freeze tag several times per week in my front yard with son Kurt and a mob of neighborhood moppets. All movement has value if it is controlled and thoughtful. Controlled and thoughtful movement is a positive stressor as well as a diminisher of negative stress.

As a practicing chiropractor, I witnessed hundreds of people not anywhere close to thoughtful and controlled body mechanics culminating in "my back went out" (neck, shoulder, or whatever body part you care to insert here). Complete misery for these people and often the same people would make the same mistakes for years. It's obvious by almost every measure that chronic inactivity is one major cause of our crippled bodies and minds. We just have to get off our couch. It only takes a second to decide to do something positive. One-second decision time.

Goal: Unbalanced

Balance training, attempting to stand or sit on an unstable surface like a BOSU ball or wobble board, or by attempting to balance on your tippy toes, is tremendous brain training. A BOSU is part of the equipment package in the Everest 70 Challenge primarily because it is so versatile. Mine is always in my living room where I write so I can stand on it and exercise my brain while simultaneously destressing. I will also stand on it periodically while writing on my stand up desk for additional brain stimulation.

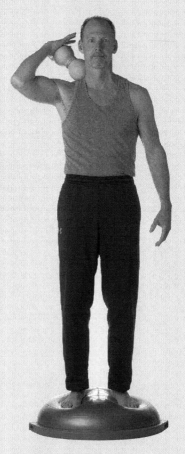

The Dopiest Exercise Mistakes Smart People Make

Failing. Blowing it. Dropping the ball. Who cares? You will blow it and so will I. As long as you reboot and reset quickly it's all just failing your way to fitness.

Too slow in rebooting? That infraction will not be tolerated dear sir or madam. This is the dopiest exercise mistake smart people make. If you have gotten out of the successful exercise habit you may have to force yourself in hitting the reset button a couple of times to get back on the beam. The following are some additional fitness faux pas.

• Too much, too soon: Doing way too many activities before your body is ready. Remember the vertical health continuum to your personal summit takes a lifetime of moments. Exercise (stimulation), then let it heal (rest, or do another unrelated play day activity).

• Not warming up: The older we get, the more time we need to spend increasing body temperature, circulation, and "greasing" the joints before launching into physical activity. See the QuickFit Base Camp routine.

• Getting out of the tone habit. Step off the wellness continuum and you regress down immediately. Sorry about this but I don't make the news I just report it. Stop the deterioration this second with a reboot or a Dyno (you will learn about this valuable technique ahead... keep reading). Yes, now. Begin by asking the two most important super-wellness questions: 1. "What do I need now?" 2. "What would serve me best now?"

• Working out alone. Mistake. All research shows people do it and keep doing it if the tribe is doing it. Even for a once/week LSD (long slow distance) day or for the three hard days or whatever works. Just include a partner or partners if possible but some zen alone time is a necessity as well. Balance.

• Bad form and holding on to cardio machines that you are not supposed to. I see this every trip to the gym. It significantly decreases the benefit of doing the exercise if you are holding on to a treadmill, for example, but worst thing is that it eliminates the brain training. This drives me crazy. Never do an exercise by mimicking another. They could be a moron. If you are unsure of an activity or how to safely perform an action, ask a staff member.

- Wrong weight. A general rule with strength and functional training is keep the repetitions between 8 and 15. If you can't do 8 reps with good form, the weight is too heavy. If you can do more than 15 it's too light. "Failure" or "AMRAP" is achieved when you can't do another repetition with good form. Shoot for this on your hard days. This is the good kind of failure.

- Crunches, sit ups, or any trunk flexion abdominal activity. I do not do crunches nor do I advocate crunches. They are not functional and they can be irritating and damaging to the lower back, mid back, and neck. My body hurts if I just think about crunches.

- People walking with hand weights should keep the weights incredibly light, nine ounces, obliterating the brain training balance aspect. I see people who believe they are getting an improved workout by carrying heavy weights while walking but in fact that ruins the natural motion of the arms.

- As a former runner with thirty years' experience, you may be surprised to hear me say that running is not the activity for everybody. There are people who are simply not built to run. Driving down the road, it is all I can do not to stop, tap runners on the shoulder, and say, "Hey Bro you would be much better off if you switched to walking,... and by the way buy ten copies of my book." Rampant imbalances, no upper body motion, aberrant leg motions, and limited stride length are just a few of the damaging problems.

- There are too many potential poor fitness techniques to comment on but I urge you to not follow blindly what you observe others doing. Do your due diligence online or with a personal trainer with whom you resonate.

Muscle Without Discipline

Most of us want to be fit for the rest of our lives. To achieve this worthy intention, we need to start slowly but tenaciously and go for it. Again, put pictures of your favorite intentional body motivation (good or bad or both) in a place where you can see it regularly, such as your journal, phone case, or blow it up in a three- by four-foot poster for your ceiling. I would also use a front and side current picture of yourself in swimsuit or underwear for added motivation.

I am now in my late fifties. The rare times I get lazy or life circumstances get in the way and I "blow it" or "fail" in fitness, I don't gain five pounds, I lose five pounds. My muscles wither and I get a "panse" (my French-Canadian ex-in-laws' word for gut). My shoulders get so bony that my lady can get a black eye if she makes the mistake of resting her head on my shoulder. This signals my motivation to Dyno and be the best I can be. I start by taking selfies in the least flattering light. Front, back, and side views. I want truth. They may be for my eyes only but that inspires me to get on the mountain and stay on it. Slipping and checking are both normal and expected so forgive yourself and move forward. Perfection is an illusion and is both unattainable and produces negative stress. Constant never ending improvement and forgiveness of self are key to toned super-fitness.

Chapter Six: Brain Train Exercise—The Fitness Dyno

Hey, it's not easy to exercise five or six days a week, year in and year out for the rest of your life. You might start skipping weeks or even months. You may throw in the towel, say the hades with it, and quit. You and I both will need a little extra motivation at times. About every seventy days or five times a year. I suggest you embrace the idea of the "Dyno." Never heard of it? Attach your climbing harness, strap in, and allow me to explain.

A Dyno High on Mount Everest

In the sport of climbing sometimes you get stuck. Really stuck. Sometimes you can't go up, down, or sideways. This is scary to say the least. Especially terrifying when you are in a precarious position as I was coming down from the summit of Everest totally exhausted and stuck in a very exposed spot on the Hillary Step with my muscles rapidly failing as slow-as-molasses ascending climbers blocked Phinjo Sherpa's and my descent. This was May 24, 2008, about 6 A.M. and we were nearly 29,000 feet in elevation with a 10,000-foot drop on one side and 7,000-foot drop on the other. We had to Dyno to stay alive. The Dyno was to bulldoze our way through an exhausted throng of wasted climbers and not hang out, be polite, and possibly die as we used up valuable oxygen, energy, and tumbled from our precarious perch. (Read more about failure and success on Mount Everest in *Lessons From Everest: 7 Powerful Steps to the Top of Your World* on Amazon or Kindle.) A Dyno is simply a dramatic active shift that changes your perspective, motivation, and results.

It's my belief that roughly five times per year there can be a lull in fitness motivation which can be in Feet, Fork, or Fun or any combination. At such times one should execute a fitness Dyno. Figure out your own plan but I suggest a dramatic change such as taking up a new sport or fitness class and do it long enough to see if it's something you will keep in your life. How about an adventure trip? Train to hike the Bright Angel Trail to Phantom Ranch at the bottom of the Grand Canyon. An adventure/obstacle race? Hook up with some buddies and learn/train together. A Dyno should be a bit beyond your present ability and should result in months of training. Haven't biked since childhood? How about buying a second hander and training for a century ride with a personal reward, if you love it, of a really cool and expensive bike? Do it right. Train to handle it. Book a yoga vacation and do their regimen. Have fun with this... doctor's orders. The point is to set an intention that marshals all your possibly dormant motivation and inspiration (Fun dimension) and involves the Feet and Fork. It is my experience since childhood that a Dyno changes everything.

I am a fan of fitness challenges as a Dyno. A fitness challenge can be preparing oneself for an event such as a 5K run, a Spartan Race, a Tuff Mudder, a hike in the White Mountains of New Hampshire, prep for a softball league, or, if you have been stationary for a long time, getting in shape to get in shape. I have used fitness challenges as successful Dynos for most of my life. As a chiropractor, I coached patients for years in a program called Creating Wellness. My practice members used the program as a Dyno to address and minimize the negative aspects of stress in all three dimensions. Our office was able to positively influence and educate many more people. I think health challenges are a natural fit for human beings. I think it simply aligns with our essence of striving for a goal. Once, at age forty, I completed a health challenge purely as a distraction from going through a divorce. It was great therapy and helped in all three dimensions.

I occasionally jet around in a rush of hotels and airports writing, speaking, and consulting. This can be a challenge for my normal super-fitness. Three breakfast buffets in three days combined by long hours, sitting on my behind, then having a cocktail will slow down any inner athlete. My normal "home" nutrition may drop to a B-, my head-space becomes a C+, my fitness peters out to a C and... my back hurts like hell. This of course results in a mini-Dyno in Feet, Fork, and Fun when I arrive home to my sanctuary.

In all life experiences, we learn a little something along the way and carry it with us forever. In health challenges, we have a net gain of fitness, understanding of ourselves, and athlete awareness that we keep forever even if we drop the ball and regress occasionally.

Hence, I introduce the Everest 70 Challenge, Chapter Ten in this book. The Feet, Fork, and Fun challenge is inspired by the seventy days required to ascend the biggest bump in the earth and the people that risk their lives attempting to climb it. Your health and mine is even more risky than a Mount Everest climb. Just look at the dis-ease statistics already shared. Seemingly a million things can go wrong in either instance and, yet, people do succeed. I want you to succeed. I want you to thrive. I want you to laugh at the mountain of adversities in the world today and march up daily to the summit. Every day is an opportunity. Why 70? Seventy days is an Everest attempt and seventy days will allow you to make concrete, measurable improvement if you choose to challenge your-self. Besides, in the Everest 70 Challenge you will not be crushed in an avalanche or die of an altitude-related catastrophe. If it's been some time since you have been active, then you can get right back on target (Dyno) while learning super-wellness concepts that will last a lifetime. If you are somewhat in shape, then experimenting with my program will add tone to your resume. If you are already a wellness lion or lioness you will be even more outrageous.

Super Fitness in 50 Words

Feet. Supple. Gentle. Functional. Fartlek. Progressive. Hard-easy, hard-easy, repeat till you're a hundred. Compete only with yourself. Brain train. Move daily. Take the stairs. Walkabout. Athletic position. Bad wedding dance. Efficiency. Ease. Progress. Easy progress. Muscle bumps. Stabilize. Six-pack. All planes all the time. Luxuriate. Sleep deeply without care. Zen.

Chapter Six: Points to Ponder

1. Bathe in protein. More in the next chapter.

2. Climb your personal Everest.

3. Cave people are sexy.

4. Dyno five times per year and don't hesitate to sprinkle mini-Dynos in as necessary.

5. Have so much fun you can't stand it.

6. Be in the best shape of your life in all three dimensions at age 40, 50, 60, 70, 80...

CHAPTER SEVEN

Fork: Eating Well

Mrs. Fufutnick wistfully to Dr. Tim: "I would love to be thin like you." Dr. Tim: "Well then drop the cookie." Mrs. Fufutnick: "No really, I would love to be thin like you." Dr. Tim: "So drop the cookie."

Salads Have More Fun

Bert was having a perfectly average Friday at his office when at the end of the 2 P.M. meeting, Sally, to much fanfare, brought in the remains of a particularly mouth-watering birthday-for-somebody cake with a dozen 4-inch by 4-inch by 4-inch pieces already cut. Dammit. He could tell at a glance it was his fave. The rich, moist white cake from the bakery down the street with the whipped cream frosting. Though only Friday, Bert had splurged on his two weekly cheat meals already and to make matters worse he had blown off his power walk the previous night. Familiar pangs of guilt coursed through Bert's body and butterflied his stomach even though he hadn't yet decided if he would indulge. Moment of truth. Should Bert (A) politely refuse the mouth-watering morsel? or (B) eat the entire mouth-watering morsel? What should a poor Bert do? What would you do?

If I had a second with Bert I would ask him how he will feel if he eats the cake while remaining alert for young Bert's verbal and nonverbal response. If the B-man was going to feel some mental and emotional pain after eating, then he shouldn't eat it. It's not worth it in the least. It's clear that his body was already doing its best to alert him to the impending downside of a poor choice. The point is this. With mindfulness (Chapter Eight, Fun) and practice it can take just a second: (1) listen carefully to your body's subtle cues then (2) ask yourself how you will feel afterward if you eat the cake or blow off the planned workout, etc. Heck, maybe a third option of carving off a quarter or a half of those monstrous pieces. Is it a big deal if you have a piece of cake when you have already had two cheat meals that week? How could it? It's just a piece of cake. In the scheme of things, it's not a blip on any screen—except that it is. It's a negative stress in all three dimensions of physical, chemical, and emotional. A negative Feet, Fork, and Fun in one fell swoop. Having that cake at that time will leave a mark especially in the Fun arena. What would happen if Bert passed apologetically on the cake, pulled out some carrots, cucumbers, and celery with a hummus dip and joined the party? That would be much more fun for Bert because the guilt, stress, and angst would not exist. Bert just got really powerful. He is the king, boss, and CEO of his Feet, Fork, and Fun. Bert wins game, set, and match. The bottom line is that the more committed you are to a healthy lifestyle, the easier and less angst-ridden these decisions become. Sometimes salad is more fun than cake!

Nutrition is at minimum 80% of our health, wellness, dis-ease, and disease prevention. Hell, it might be 95%. At any rate the vast majority of our life, tone, and human potential derive from what we do, and do not, put into our mouths.

Chapter Seven: Brain Train Exercise

Grow something. Grow stuff at your crib. Get dirt under your fingernails. Save money and get healthier by growing things at home. You don't have to cultivate huge vegetable and pollinator gardens unless that's your dream. Use a patch of dirt or a couple of containers on your deck and put in some tomatoes or herbs for your salad. If you can't do any of that then get on www.mercola.com and buy the Sprout Doctor Starter Kit and grow your own salads on your kitchen counter.

Paleosity: Eat Like a Mediterranean Caveman

"Paleo": Eating plan that resembles our Paleolithic hunter-gatherer ancestry. Good quality protein including lean meats, poultry, and fish. Vegetables, fruits, good fats, and nuts recommended. Dairy products, grains, and legumes (beans) not included.

"Mediterranean": The Mediterranean nutrition plan involves eating primarily plant-based foods such as fruits and vegetables, whole grains, legumes, and nuts. Lean protein such as fish and poultry over red meat. Using herbs and spices to season foods. Using healthy fats such as olive oil rather than butter. Red wine is consumed regularly but moderately.

There are similarities to the above two plans but I have used author privilege to take the best and leave the rest, plus life is just not worth living without a good Cabernet. The result: Paleosity.

Why, yes, I did make up the word Paleosity. Want to live longer and stronger? My nutritional vision is to incorporate a combination of Mediterranean and Paleo nutrition into your world to nourish your buff body and mind. I call it Paleosity because it is not as strict a nutritional regimen as hard core Paleolithic lifestyle as promulgated by Dr. Loren Cordain, Robb Wolf (see appendix for bibliography), and others, but retains much of the benefits. A hybrid, if you will.

In my research and experience, Paleosity is the best plan to feed your 70 trillion cells, reduce inflammation and dis-ease, and achieve an optimum weight by promoting natural fat loss with muscle retention. Additional benefits include optimizing energy, vitality, sleep quality, and mental acuity. It also has enough variety to satiate most palates.

My purpose is not to confuse the message with all the nutrition facts available, but to provide the meat and sweet potatoes necessary to get well and stay well. You can research further by perusing the resources for further study in the Appendix while you snack on some raw almonds.

Dr. Tim's Paleosity Plan

Eat These	Don't Eat These	Ok, but just a smidge
Fish, poultry, meat, eggs	Dairy products	Greek yogurt
Vegetables	Cereals, breads, grains	Red Wine
Good Fats	Refined sugars	Some beans
Organic coffee, teas, water	Soda, juices, sports drinks	Some cheeses

See the Chapter Seven section of the Appendix for a handful of mouth-watering Paleosity recipes.

Why Diets Hate You and Want to Kill You

Have you been on a diet? Have you been on a thousand diets? If "diets" "worked" there would be no need for a second or third or one hundredth go at the diet smörgåsbord. I do not want to disrespect the multitudes of folk who are going out there and kicking and screaming to improve themselves and certainly most action is better than no action at all but there is a simpler, less mentally and physically taxing, less inflaming, and truer to our nature way. It's lifestyle. Find a sane road map and work it forever. Tweak this plan as your experience, education, and research progresses. I know, I know, easier said than done in our celebrity weight loss obsessed, Twitter-dominated, fast-paced diet information snippet world but the truth is the truth.

Once again, I honor, respect, and applaud folks who are committed to making a positive change in their physical, chemical, and emotional world but I propose a different paradigm. I propose the concept of life-style change because that mindset and attitude will make the necessary evolution from the same-old, same-old of American "health" or lack thereof to a new world of vitality and true wellness. Lifestyle means a program that the perpetrator of wellness maintains forever. Not for 70 days, not for 365 days, not for 3,650 days, but the entirety of days.

Yessiree, a failed and overused concept in the lexicon of nutrition and wellness is the idea of the diet. Nothing would make me happier than to never hear the word again or better yet hear of anyone going on a diet, staying on a diet, stopping the diet, etc. The reader will never hear me touting a diet. When I begrudgingly use the word in a speech or here and there in this book I am referring to a lifestyle improvement not an inherently short-term paroxysm. I don't like diets for many reasons but here are two:

- I dislike the first three letters in the word "diet."

- They don't work. Diets don't work because they are short-term band-aid approaches. Even if many people "succeed" in their minds and lose some weight, it adds nothing to their overall wellness or health. It's also been shown that the yo-yo effect of dieting (losing and gaining the same 20 to 200 pounds over and over and over) is damaging to the body and depressing for the mind.

Paleosity, the author's nutritional Fork plan, is lifestyle oriented not short-term or diet-ish. Exercise, nutrition, and head space mindfulness recommendations featured in this book are also designed to be performed for life. A lifestyle is one of healthful and sustained health habits for a lifetime and not a short-sighted, temporary fix.

I used to eat a lot of natural foods until I learned that some people die of natural causes.—Unknown

Dr. Tim's Top Ten (plus one) Titillating Tidbits of Tone: Fork

1. Consume plant-based foods as they have a high nutrient-to-calorie ratio as a main focus. Eat a colorful variety of vegetables and fruits along with nuts and seeds.

2. Consume the most nutrients and the least additives by eating food that is whole, fresh, seasonal, local, unrefined, and not processed. This is way easier than it was even a year ago.

3. For protein eat clean. Clean means wild caught, grass fed, free range. Again, this is way easier than it was even a year ago.

4. Consume healthy fats. Choose essential fats from whole food sources such as nuts, seeds, avocados, olives, and coconut. See my Fork Matrix coming up next.

5. Eat two to five meals per day depending on activity level and goals. For most of us two or three tops are enough.

6. Life is what happens between the vacations, holidays, and special events. Pay attention and consume correctly for your (intentional) life.

7. Moments matter. When at crossroads, make a positive choice while ignoring a negative and reap self-esteem and super-wellness as a result.

8. Plan ahead with meals and snacks to eliminate last second unhealthy choices.

9. Minimize exposure by skin, breathing, ingestion, or proximity to chemicals and toxins including prescriptions, cleaners, additives, and yard, shop, and under-the-kitchen-counter chemicals.

10. Drink water. Minimize sugar, salt (Himalayan sea salt sparingly), and flour or anything made with it.

11. Don't despair. Enjoy two cheat meals/week. For example, if I want a big fat dessert at a restaurant that counts as one cheat. If I want the Mediterranean pizza at Boston Neck Pizza that is my second cheat meal of the week.

It's what you do most of the time that counts.—The Author

The Fork Matrix

I am not interested in cooking at all. Never have been. It's just not my thing. Probably relates to my self-diagnosed ADHD. I would much rather go out and have an adventure than spend time slaving away in my kitchen. I am the classic eat-to-live rather than live-to-eat dude. Here's the thing though, I am very, very interested in having the best nutrition possible to fuel my lifestyle. How can I possibly balance both? How can I find a non-pain-in-the-glutes, non-demanding, easy-breezy minimal effort way to get the best Paleosity nutrition into my blood stream and 70 trillion cells? The answer: The Fork Matrix. The way to instantly have available over 35,000 different awesome meals. Simply pick one from each column. The Fork Matrix means dinner doesn't have to repeat for over 100 years, or breakfast, lunch, and dinner not repeating for over 30 years.

Protein	Vegetables	Spices	Fats/oils
Bacon	Broccoli	Ginger	Olive
Buffalo Steaks/burg	Kale	Garlic	Coconut
Chicken Breast	Chard	Allspice	Almond
Chicken Sausage	Endive	Cinnamon	Macadamia
Ground Beef	Fennel	Turmeric	Pecan
Lamb Chops	Onions	Cilantro	Walnut
Pork Loin	Brussel Sprouts	Cumin	Hazelnut
Pork Ribs	Cabbage	Red Curry	Lard
Salmon	Asparagus	Basil	Sesame
Shrimp	Celery	Oregano	Pistachio
Stew Meat	Peppers-Red	Garam Masala	Avocado
Tuna	Peppers-Green	Salt and pepper	Flaxseed
Turkey	Carrots	Lemon Zest	Bacon fat
Venison	Sweet Potato	Chile Powder	

Let food be thy medicine and medicine be thy food.—Hippocrates

Health Without Discipline

Discipline is overrated for super-wellness. Screw discipline.

In Feet, Fork, and Fun, we mentally check and recheck multiple times throughout the day and simply make health choices consistent with our goals. In case of quandary, launch into the STOP method to avoid the most common causes of failure in any worthwhile endeavor: C.R.A.P. (complacency, rationalization, apathy, and procrastination).

Use the STOP method to avoid mindless habits that do not serve your body or mind. The acronym STOP in the nutritional realm results in either making a positive choice or avoiding a negative nutritional choice or both. Our friend Bert could used this on his Friday afternoon at the office when the devil incarnate showed up.

S = Stop.

T = Take a deep breath.

O = Observe what is happening in your environment and in your mind.

P = Proceed to Succeed.

The STOP method is an easy antidote to reboot into the present moment and avoid choices that lower self-esteem and take you away from your intentions. If STOP doesn't do the trick, then ask the two big questions: "What would serve me best now?" and "What do I need now?" (Not "What do I want?" but "What do I need?").

Shop for Muscle and Return the Flab

While living with locals in France and Germany a few years ago, I realized that the reason they had little tiny refrigerators was that they had access to fresh food all day right down the street. If Americans have to go to the farmer's market on a Saturday morning and do major food shopping Sunday afternoon, for example, then that works, but what I am saying is make it easy and efficient so you have plenty of time to play tag with the kids or watch the Sox on a Sunday afternoon.

Type 2 diabetes runs in your family because nobody runs in your family.—Unknown

Unless you love the lost time and hassle of multiple food shopping trips, why not get it all done in one fell swoop. I like Sundays for this but do whatever works for your situation. Unless you live in Europe and can get fresh, awesome food every day at the end of the street, it is best to do it once a week or, at most, twice a week. Since my home is at the end of a long driveway deep in the woods, I have a goal of the truck leaving the driveway not more than once/day or seven times/week because it's a time suck. The most awesome days are when the car doesn't leave the driveway at all. To reduce emotional stress, look at your time sucks and remove them. More on emotional stress reduction in the next chapter, Fun.

Remember the term sarcopenia (muscle wasting) from the last chapter? What you do or don't eat helps or hinders your lifelong sarcopenia battle. Since muscle clears glucose (blood sugar), and boosts metabolism, your properly functioning body consumes its own fat. Muscle, therefore is your bestie. In other words, the more muscle you have the less belly and saddlebags hang off... automatically.

To win the sarcopenia war it's of prime importance to have a deeply fulfilling relationship with protein.

Put the Pro in Protein

1. RDA (recommended daily allowance) for 135-lb person is 200 grams; with exercise that RDA goes up to 660 grams.

2. Have some protein first thing in the morning and throughout the day.

3. Must exercise and eat properly to minimize sarcopenia.

4. Protein is driven by leucine (an amino acid building block of protein). Read labels as you need at least 2.2 grams/day of leucine.

5. Sugar is bad news for sarcopenia prevention.

6. Eating carbohydrates at night before bed leaches protein.

7. High protein helps you lose weight, increases libido, promulgates sleep, lowers total cholesterol, raises good cholesterol, stabilizes blood sugar, and lowers inflammation.

Liquid Muscles (and Vegetables)

I love muscle shakes. My muscle shakes always have (mega) vegetables, fruit, and protein powder within a base liquid, usually unsweetened juice. I like shakes so much I have two blenders in case one peters out. Muscle shakes are an easy, nutritious way to get additional greens if you are not yet in the habit. Toss a handful of raw spinach in a blender and you will not even know it is there. I have at least one per day, and drinking a shake is a great way to drink a meal or repair muscle after a workout. I like vanilla or chocolate Pure Power Protein from Dr. Mercola.

Muscle Shake Matrix

Blend your choice of ingredients from each category.
Makes two 16-oz shakes.

Base: 2 to 2.5 cups water, unsweetened juice, almond, or coconut beverage.	
Fruit: 1 to 1.5 cups bananas, mangoes, peaches, cherries, apples, fresh or frozen berries, pineapple chunks, dates	Vegetables: 1 to 1.5 cups spinach, kale, avocado, chard, cucumber, chopped beets
Protein: vanilla or chocolate but other flavors available	Other cool stuff: 1 teaspoon for aromatics and/or 3 tablespoons seeds or nut butter, cinnamon, ginger, almond butter, flaxseed, chia seed, vanilla extract, mint, cacao powder, honey, hemp seeds, pure maple sugar, sunflower seeds

Fork Super Fitness in 50-ish Words

Choose whole, unprocessed, unrefined, unmodified super foods that can be hunted or gathered. Shop local responsible producers. Eat animals, eggs, seafood, vegetables, fruits, nuts, and seeds. Eat fats from pastured animals, seafood, coconut, avocado, and olives. Drink water. Seek nutrient-dense super foods including fermented vegetables and beverages and forget diets and gimmicks. Pretend the modern supermarket does not exist.

Chapter Seven: Points to Ponder

1. Eat like a caveperson in Florence: Paleosity.

2. My plate is healthier than the fed's plate.

3. Nutrition is for a lifetime and not a diet for Bob and Martha's wedding next June.

4. Eat and exercise for muscle and fat loss takes care of itself.

5. Have a V8-powered turbo diesel super charged 500-horse power blender... or two.

6. *"Paleosity: 100% paleo... 80% of the time."*—*The Author*

CHAPTER EIGHT

Fun: Thinking Well

The soul should always stand ajar, ready to welcome the ecstatic experience.—Emily Dickenson

Winning the Game of Mind

"The natural state of your mind is like a drunk monkey," says sports psychologist Michael Gervais, PhD. Always looking for the new shiny object, overly curious, all over the place, and naturally distracted, our monkey mind needs to get back to the present. With a wee bit of discipline, we can do just that. A simple activity is to focus intently on mundane daily events. When you get into your car, focus on the sound of ignition and your engine for example. When you walk into work, focus on crossing the threshold, taking a deep breath, and having one thought of your work life intention. The plan is to clear the drunk monkey mind and be fully present and by default: effective. When you walk into your home, stop, breathe, "intend," and really BE at home with your family.

The Three Types of Fun (and why all are important)

Who doesn't like fun? I'll bet 99% of people agree that they are totally down for fun. However, I expect blank stares when the same people are asked, "What is fun?" I submit that there are actually three types of fun.

Type 1 Fun: In the moment fun. This is the typical type of fun and what most people think of as "fun." Examples: Going to a party with friends. A relaxing stroll in the park. You most likely don't want the perfect skiing or beach day to end.

Type 2 Fun: Enjoyment in retrospect. Running a half marathon. A long backpacking trip in sideways rain. During the actual event you could really be hating it but, as time goes by, you have wistful fond memories of your suffering. The funny thing is this type of fun creates some awesome stories.

Type 3 Fun: This is the no fun, fun. The type of fun you wouldn't wish on your worst enemy. Examples include climbing Mount Everest, Shackleton crossing the Antarctic, your car breaking down in the middle of the desert or whitewater rafting the Wolf River in Wisconsin when your two-person raft flips and you are breathing air under the overturned raft tenuously hanging on by one hand while smashing into rocks going over Pissmire Falls before losing your shoe with your car key on it and very nearly letting your buddy "Gunman" shoot out your hatchback lock with a 9-mm. (Not that any of this happened to Jay and me.) "Failed" experiences and risk of injury or death are hard to think of as "fun" but these become pivotal learning experiences that allow us to appreciate when things are on the straight and narrow. Sometimes Type 3 fun happens when we least expect it and later we can look back, crack a smile, and celebrate our fortitude.

I started this book by proclaiming "This book is for losers." My hope is that everyone embraces their inner loser... but only, only, only if you see failure for what it truly is: the fertilizer of success, positive change, growth, and learning.

There's always a second chance, it's called tomorrow.—Unknown

I'm not sure anybody learns anything from success, but I for one have learned a ton from the grueling preparation of worthwhile endeavors and mostly from the painful sting of screwing things up.

May your days be filled with Type 1 Fun, your memories chock full of Type 2 Fun, and your judgment based on Type 3 Fun.

If a man insisted on always being serious, and never allowing himself a bit of fun and relaxation, he would go mad or become unstable without knowing it.—Herodotus

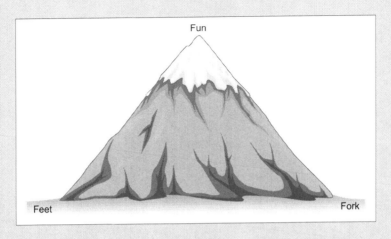

It might be just me, but I am not into any process if I am not going to have fun. Being healthy and knowing innately that you are living the wellness lifestyle and making great choices is more than fun. It's more like Fun, Fun, Fun! Being out of shape is not fun. Having energy and the self-satisfaction of eating well is really fun. Disappointing myself by eating poorly when I know I can do better is no fun.

Negative stress in the emotional dimension is most assuredly not fun. Learning, working, experimenting, adventuring, guilt-free luxuriating are Fun, Fun, Fun. Chronic wellness has to be fun if you are going to keep your life moving and grooving for 120 years.

When I say "fun," I am referring to the Type 1, warm, feel-good sensation of self-satisfaction that comes with following through in any personal or business endeavor. It's the warm fuzzies of a job well done. In our health example those warm fuzzy feelings are associated with moving the ball forward (ascending the wellness continuum). Progressing on any plan is fun, and sadly for many people it is a rare occurrence to feel good and have fun. I urge everyone to give it a go. If Fun is not in your present experience then change some things around. Put on your big girl or big boy pants and figure it out. Dyno!

In rock climbing a Dyno is when you leap for a hold that is out of reach. It's a no-holds-barred, feet flying, go-for-it, damn-the-torpedoes move. Remember this in terms of the Fun dimension the next time you feel stuck in your life. Often when ascending a vertical rock wall there are times when it appears there is no place to go. Scary. What I have learned is that if you inch up just a smidge—not even an inch at times—the whole world changes. Opportunities that once were invisible are now obvious. Never forget this.

Brain Fun

Your brain needs learning for sustenance. Learning is brain food. To be super-well you must be learning. Not simply traditional schooling but brain stimulation to age 120 and perhaps beyond. Learning is brain exercise. Different brain exercise than the Bad Wedding Dance or Super Brain Yoga but brain fitness nonetheless. The brain is "plastic" and mold-able even into old age and needs stimulation, just like a muscle, to remain healthy. In fact, there are entire medical journals related to the science of neuroplasticity. Learning and mindfulness are that stimulation. But the brain is even more important than the body, isn't it? It's the computer system of the body so it needs more attention than the body. "What's that you say, Dr. Tim? My brain needs even more exercise than my body? And now I have to meditate for hours, too?" Yes, the brain needs attention and, no, you don't have to meditate or remain mindful for hours. It needn't be an extra line on your to do list or another item on your intention card but to be super-well the computer needs input.

Brain Dynos

"Challenge." Doesn't the word just sound cool? Challenge is learning for the brain. What happens if you don't move the TV room furniture once in a while to clean? You have dust, dead moths, cat hair, doggie presents, and food objects left over from the last Red Sox World Series celebration. If you don't challenge the brain it stagnates, gets stale, and gets "dusty." The solution? Dyno that thang. Dyno means shake it up, change your mind, and change your life. A Dyno is brain fartlek. Challenge it. Learn. Examples: travel, crossword puzzles, chess, cards, word problems, numbers games, jigsaw puzzles, take up a musical instrument, learn to read music, study maps, read everything in sight, write letters, take courses, teach others, be social, fight loneliness at all times, fix something broken around the house or on your car, take a painting course, write your journal, dance, date provocative people or—even better—marry one, race sailboats... there are endless possibilities but the key is challenge.

Q: "Is TV brain exercise?"

A: "No, TV is mind candy to sell you stuff you don't need while you rot in your recliner."

Knowledge is good.—Col. Faber (*Animal House* opening scene)

Chapter Eight: Brain Train Exercise— Four Lifestyle Changes That Protect the Brain

1. Move the body. Physical activity reduces cognitive decline and grows certain regions of the brain that tend to shrink during aging. Check the box. Done deal. See Chapter Five, Feet.

2. Feed the heart to feed the brain. Reducing the risk of heart disease has very strong evidence of brain benefits. A Paleosity lifestyle will reduce inflammation, hypertension, high blood fats, cholesterol, obesity, and Type 2 diabetes. Check the box. Done deal. See Chapter Seven, Fork.

3. Learn, challenge, and Dyno. Interacting with the world intellectually over a lifetime has been shown to lead to better cognitive health in old folks. Check the box. Done deal. See this chapter, Fun.

4. Sleep. Some studies have found a relationship between poor sleep habits and brain decline and Alzheimer's. Let's deal with snooze right now.

My former chiropractic college roomie Dr. Phil (not that Dr. Phil) has a sister who is a Silicon Valley Tech superstar. She most recently started a health technology company and was collecting data on the most searched health problems or concerns to people in Western society. She expected diabetes or Alzheimer's or arthritis or diet but the results shocked her: the most searched health problem of our Western world was "How do I get to sleep?" Sleep is most definitely a "Feet" subject but I decided to include it in this chapter because it seems to fit better with the brain discussion and "there ain't no fun without sleep."

Twelve Ways to Get and Stay Asleep

I refer to the search for healthy, recuperative, and healing sleep as sleep hygiene. I refrain from repeating the litany of disorders and diseases both physical and mental that result from poor sleep as I am sure you have heard them all. Let me just say that 25% of Americans have occasional insomnia and 10% have chronic insomnia. Let's get right to fixing the sleep conundrum by instituting sleep hygiene into your life.

1. Go to bed and arise at the same time every day, 7 days/week. It's all about establishing rhythms.

2. Complete darkness needed. Put tape over the lights on your smoke detector, use blackout shades, or sleep with a comfy eye mask.

3. Don't eat within an hour of sleep and, as noted in Chapter Seven, grains and sugars especially suck for you at night. But protein and some fruit or berries can be helpful for sleep hormone production. Also, caffeine and alcohol both inhibit sleep hygiene. Prescription and over-the-counter drugs should be minimized to what is absolutely necessary.

4. No devices or TV in the bedroom. If you must have your phone handy use a free app such as SleepBot or Sleep Cycle.

5. If your mind races when you lie in bed, have a journal close by to jot notes. This serves to download your junk.

6. Utilize "paleo sleep" by darkening your evening an hour before you crash. Regress to the preindustrial night and eliminate artificial light. This cues your body's melatonin pump.

7. Minimize fluid intake 2 hours before bed if you get up routinely to tinkle.

8. A leisurely hot bath, shower, or hot tub is relaxing before beddy-bye.

9. Make sure you have a mattress, sheets, and pillows that are conducive to your sleep hygiene. Sleep is our body's recuperative one-third of our entire life.

10. Holistic doc Andrew Weil says he can knock you out in a minute by performing the "4-7-8" technique derived from yoga. Breathe in for 4 seconds, hold for 7, exhale forcefully for 8. Repeat three times. Weil says, with practice, you can produce an altered state of consciousness. Cool.

11. Cool the room to 65 degrees and wear socks if the toes get cold. Neurologist and sleep expert Charles Winter reminds us to not "try" to fall asleep; rather, perform an action in your mind like mowing your lawn. The brain can only do one function at a time so usually you'll be out before you finish mental mowing even once.

12. The recommendations in Feet and Fork as well as this chapter, Fun, form a balanced physical, chemical, and emotional dynamic "ease" (as opposed to dis-ease) for the reader serious about health. In other words, following Feet and Fork protocol benefits Fun and by default, sleep. Night, night.

Winning the Head Game of Health With Empowered Mindfulness

Empowered mindfulness is utilizing your powerful intentions to make esoteric human ideals meaningful in the real world. Empowered mindfulness is the foundation of becoming the highest potential, best version of yourself as a human being. The following items make up the "7 Powerful Steps to the Top of Your World" as described in my first book *Lessons From Everest*. Together, the seven steps define empowered mindfulness:

1. What's your Everest? Read: what is your mission, talent, destiny... your purpose?

2. Love your work.

3. Enjoy the ride because life is the ride.

4. Hope: a shred is all you need.

5. Thank your way to the top.

6. Pay attention: awareness is now.

7. Find, reconnect, or modify your metaphorical Everest. In other words, once you climb one Everest, you must define and work toward your next Everest.

Number 1 is mandatory on your intention card. Define it and redefine it. No worries if you define and redefine purpose for the rest of your life. Most people never do it once.

Descartes' Error

Let's establish that there is a mind–body connection, contrary to what the French philosopher Rene Descartes postulated in the 1700s. He was the dude who said that mind and body were separate and distinct.

Can I prove to you that mind and body are one? Ok, close your eyes and sit back. Come on, do it! Take a deep breath and imagine this scenario. I am selecting a very plump, very ripe lemon. I am rolling the lemon around my granite counter to break open the internal juice cells of the lemon so the lemon nearly explodes as I cut it in half. Now I ask you to hold out your hand as I place half of the cut lemon in your hand. The juice pools in your palm and drips copiously over the floor. I ask you to bring the lemon half to your lips and take a large bite. The juice explodes into your mouth and out into the room. Ok, now stop and open your eyes. Let me ask, "Are you salivating? Is your mouth full of saliva?" Mine is just from typing this passage. Here's another question: "Do you actually have a lemon in your mouth?" No, but wait a minute, why is your body functioning as if there was? Because... there is a mind–body connection. This insight means our mind and body are both on our success team. We can influence our mind so we had better do it correctly by utilizing the empowered mindfulness protocol.

Manage Your Moments

When are your weak moments? Are there moments in your day when your resolve is a little weak? Who are you with at these times or are you alone? Pay attention to those times when you have blown it in the past. Not only nutritionally when Sarah always brings chemically cream filled donuts at 10 A.M. but physically when you could be taking the stairs rather than the elevator (this Sarah character is a sugar addict, apparently). What can you do to shake up these moments? Have a protein shake? Eat a handful of almonds? Take five big gulps of water? Or do you need a few minutes by yourself for some deep oxygenating breaths and mini meditation? Get out of your chair and walk around your desk 10 times? Do something that is the highest priority rather than the easy item on the list. Is there something you have been putting off that needs to be confronted? Fun, fun, fun is the payoff, remember? Also, remember to continuously ask the two life changing questions: "What do I need?" and "What would serve me best now?" Ask until age 120 then you can stop awhile.

One-Second Awesome

This is the magic moment of self-satisfaction that you are proactively following through on your plans for a better, healthier life. Guess what? It increases your health greatly to feel great. How great is that? Alert! Alert! Alert! Here is the super powerful secret that, one more time, should make you instantly awesome if you are not already. When you make a good one-second, in the moment, choice in any of the three dimensions of Feet, Fork, and Fun, then you automatically get benefit in the other dimensions. Sweeeeet.

For example, if you decide to walk at lunch instead of sit on your blutarski, obviously that has the benefit in the Feet aspect of your wellness, but the benefits are many in the Fork dimension by aiding digestion, utilization of food to muscle, etc. and additionally exercise benefits the Fun aspect of your wellness greatly by feeling self-satisfied about owning your power and wellness follow through. This is a big picture item and it should give you additional confidence that you will be successful. To further bombard you with this key point, if you string some clean and healthy meals together, you generate Fun in the psychological dimension but in the physical (Feet) realm you are feeding your 70 trillion cells properly, building muscle, burning fat, increasing natural immunity, and a thousand million other functions that you will never know but don't worry because your innate intelligence does and it is on the job 24/7 365 from womb to tomb.

The realization that a one-second good decision in any one dimension pays huge health benefits in the remaining two dimensions should be a shout-from-the-rooftop moment. This may seem like a simple point but the sad truth is that most folks do not participate in this most simple aspect of a healthy lifestyle. Additionally, the idea that every good habit performed facilitates a healing effect in other apparently disparate human dimensions should take some pressure and anxiety out of the process of ascending the wellness continuum. Don't over think it. After all, it's not rocket surgery.

> *Character consists of what you do on the third and fourth tries.*
> —James Michener

Scare Yourself Daily

"Adventure only happens if the outcome is unknown," said climbing buddy Rob Scott while we were stuck in a collapsing tent at 11,000 feet on Denali in Alaska while in the midst of a 66-inch blizzard over three days. Here's the good news: you don't have to climb a mountain and freeze your butt off to have adventure. Applying for a new job, going to a party where you don't know anybody, comforting a friend in grief, updating a resume, giving a speech, raising a child, confronting a loved one in an intimate relationship, or hitting the reset button on your fitness are all worthy adventures.

I have found that throwing yourself out there, on the mercy of the world, and attempting something that scares you, creates a personal culture of bravery and personal growth. While certainly a boon to our own self-esteem just think of the great lessons for those watching you like your family and close friends. Accept the one-second wellness mantle of role model to help others succeed at health. Helping others is great for ourselves as much as for others. Service to others is a deep human need that should be fed and watered. What if you try something and fall flat on your face in so-called failure? This will happen. It has certainly happened with me on numerous occasions. Actually, I hope it happens the rest of my life because that will mean that I am out there kicking and screaming, evolving, and taking chances. One of the great wisdoms is the realization that so-called bad experiences are the greatest life learning tools (and make great stories later in life).

I remember backpacking trips or climbing expeditions where everything went to hell. We ran out of food or there was no water and we resorted to sucking water out of moose prints while walking on delaminated, duct taped boots. It's funny that these trips are the ones

I remember most vividly and taught me the most. So get out there, faithful readers, and live your life as a series of daily adventures. Just remember the duct tape.

I never lose. I only win or learn.—Anonymous

Keep Your Mind in Line with the Divine So You Feel Fine

Have you heard that meditation is good for you? Have you read a book or two, seen it on Oprah, or heard a speaker say that mindfulness is important for success in life? The subject is well researched and supported by science but people make it too complicated. As a self-diagnosed ADHD dude, I myself have made it too complicated. Mindfulness means paying attention, on purpose, to the present moment, without judgment. That's it. The practice of mindfulness allows us to "fall awake" to our life while rediscovering that there is more right about us than wrong at any given moment. I think of mindfulness practice (practiced regularly not just reading about it) as grad school in the art of living. In turn, mindfulness cultivates intimacy with the "now" or the ordinary. The comedian Flip Wilson used to have a bit as the pastor of the Church of "What's Happening Now." You are the budding pastor of your "What's Happening Now," just as I am with mine.

Failure: The fertilizer of success.—The Author

One-Second Reboot

As a child, I was brought up Quaker and a major part of attending meeting on Sundays was sitting in silence for an hour. No minister or priest. Squirmy for me as an overly energetic young boy but good brain training. Silence is a very powerful meditative experience but it doesn't have to take an hour. You can do it in a minute if you consciously intend it. You can do a quick version if you mindfully take a deep breath and "be" whatever you are doing and wherever you are just as long as what you are doing doesn't involve iPads or TV. I believe that meditation happens also while being active such as raking the leaves, digging a hole, or out on a walk. As a matter of fact, the more you use your conscious mind (i.e., an accountant with his nose in the numbers or a manager managing minions), the more routine or mindless work (cleaning the house or weeding the garden) is required to offset the stress. Mindfulness can be cultivated in two ways: formally, through taught meditation techniques, some of which I will share later in this chapter; and, secondly, and more informally, by simply noticing the moments of our lives. A one-second reboot.

Can you see the integrated perfect connection of the three dimensions Feet, Fork, and Fun? That focusing on improvement in one area positively impacts all? Positively impacting all areas = tone.

Reboot Rituals That Resonate

Don't have time to meditate, you say? Well, you are missing the point. It's not about time.

Mindfulness is paying attention, on purpose, in the present moment, non-judgmentally... as if your life depended on it. Because it does.
—Dr. Jon Kabat-Zinn

With this definition, by this master, meditation/mindfulness can happen while doing or not doing anything. Many of the most successful people on the planet make regular time to meditate even if they do not call it meditation—even if it is 10 silent minutes locked in your bathroom. Ohm on the throne.

The STOP method of rebooting is perfect for a one-second meditation. Like the pattern interruption of STOP in the Feet and Fork dimensions, the STOP method of meditation is instant. It's a great way to check yourself and proceed with your desires and climb of tone. Remember STOP stands for Stop, Take a breath, Observe, and Proceed (to succeed).

Do you have some reboot rituals of your own to share? Drop an email of your fave reboot to the author at tim@drtimwarren.com.

Ten Mindfulness Tips in Real Life

1. When you first wake up in the morning, take a moment to observe how your body feels. What sounds do you hear? How does the warmth and softness of the blankets feel? Then make the bed, read your 3 × 5 intention card, and place it on your pillow.

2. Observe the sounds, smells, and feel of the shower and the bathroom.

3. When eating breakfast and/or savoring coffee, shut off any radio, TV, or electronics and savor the taste and texture. What's outside today? What's new out there, I wonder?

4. While driving, notice what's different. There is always something different in construction, plant growth, or activity. Take different routes and explore.

5. When walking between meetings or errands, notice how your body feels, notice any sense of rush in body or mind. While still getting things done, feel your feet beneath you and pay attention to any tension that may creep in.

6. When interacting with other people, really listen to them and give them the gift of full attention and connecting with them in a genuine manner.

7. At work, sit minimally and move subtly all day. Walk when you can and stretch when you can and stand on an unstable surface like a BOSU, if possible.

8. When multitasking, remember that you can only do one thing at a time so concentrate on that then move to the next thing. Devote attention to one thing only. Practice.

9. While walking with the family and/or the dog, take the time to notice the world around you. There is always something different. Explore with all your senses. After all, that's what Buster is doing.

10. Before bedding down, reflect on the day. What went right and what went wrong? Feel the blessings of both. How might you attend to your intentions differently mañana? Read your intention card and place it on the nightstand. ZZZZZZ

White Noise

Dr. Dennis Perman is a chiropractor, coach, and friend. I first heard of his white noise meditation several years ago in a lecture, forgot about it, then started using it again. I feel the exercise is one of the simplest and easiest ways to bring the benefits of mindfulness meditation into your life. Inevitably when we are sitting comfortably, extraneous thoughts enter our heads. My nose itches. My right big toe hurts. I forgot to take out the garbage. I should be making that phone call. Did Big Papi hit a home run last night? I should be at work. I wonder what the kids are doing. Blah, blah, blah...

The white noise exercise means you quiet your mind while creating your own white noise. When an extraneous thought weasels its way into your brain while attempting to be zen, take the last word of said thought and repeat it and repeat it. For example, I should be raking the lawn... lawn... lawn... lawn... lawn... lawn...

Repeating the last word turns the meaningless into mastery of meditation with practice. The practice of mindfulness results in finding the space within the space.

Don't like that method or need some variety? Here are four more awesome rebooting meditations from a series of research studies at the University of California at San Diego.

1. Body focus. Lying on the floor without a pillow, focus your attention on the top of your head. Move downward to each body part until you reach your toes. Takes anywhere from 3 to 40 minutes.

2. Standing yoga. Try poses like the tree (standing on one leg with the sole of your other foot against your inner thigh) and the chair (a sustained two-legged squat, as if seated in an imaginary chair). Hold if you can for 20 seconds and progress to 3 minutes.

3. Sitting meditation. Concentrate on the in-and-out of your breathing then widen your attention to include sensations like the pressure of your body on the chair or floor. As extraneous thoughts enter your mind, observe them but don't react or judge them. Perform this daily for at least 10 minutes.

4. Breath connection. Sit in a comfortable position on the floor or a chair and focus on breathing without changing it at all. Count 10 breaths. Repeat. Continue for 5 minutes initially then go longer.

5. Another? I love the aforementioned Super Brain Yoga activity for brain balance, de-stressing, and mindfulness.

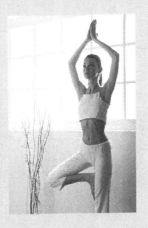
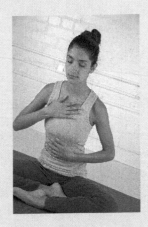

My Cave or Yours?

Remember our DNA ancestry with 50,000-year-old cave peeps? That means we are mostly identical to our spear throwing brethren except for the accouterments and habits of the modern world. Even though the cavemen had wondrous IKEA-designed caves back in the day, they were known to spend more time outside in nature than the cave people of today. People are so busy that they forget or choose other activities rather than taking that walk or packing for that picnic, all the while our DNA essence demands for us to be outside. DNA demands us being in the green, on the water, in the mountains, or in the desert. Simply to be in nature. We did not evolve in glass but in grass. Nature comforts us and I can promise that spending time in nature will soothe the modern savage beast even if you get outside only a few hours per month. Play is another thing lacking. If you watch children play you can see imagination and present time consciousness in their eyes. Where did we lose that? Don't ponder too long—just grab the fam, get outside, and start playing. No fam? Find your tribe of like-minded crazies. Check meetup.com or start your own Meetup group. Start a new life chapter by playing.

We did not evolve in glass but in grass.—The Author

How Dirty Feet Keep You Healthy

Take your togs off and get your feet in the dirt. Have a beach nearby? Walk it barefoot as often as you can. Grass? Great. Walk on it barefoot as often as you can. Dirt, grass, sand... the earth grounds you in more ways than one. The idea of grounding is that skin contact with the earth depolarizes the electromagnetic forces that build up in our bodies due to our modern lifestyle. I have heard that Tour de France riders would sleep with a special sleeping bag with their feet in the dirt so they could detox while snoozing between stages. Even better if you live on a coast and have easy access to salt water beaches. The negative ions of the ocean combined with barefoot walking is a cocktail of de-stress. I can sometimes walk barefoot on Narragansett Town Beach in Rhode Island into December.

I Dare You

Are you nuts enough to do this? Bond with your cave dude or cave dudette essence with the following activity at least once/year. Get some basic equipment and all the food and water you need and go out by yourself in a tent in the wilderness with no books, devices, and nobody to talk to. A journal and pen only. This would be life changing to know that you can be alone and at peace with your past, present, and future. Christ spent time in the wilderness just as the Buddha spent time under the Bodhi Tree. For many, maybe even most, what frightens us is not the grizzly bear but the demons that lurk in our own mind.

The reason that awareness of awareness is so powerful is that it immediately puts me in touch with a dimension of myself that knows that all things are possible.—Ken Keis, PhD

Fun in 100 Words (plus a few more).

Have fun, be fun, make up fun. Be aware. Stay awake. Bow. Feel. Sing. Create and envision. Let go, forgive, and accept. Work, serve, and contribute. Practice tai chi. Listen, learn, and inquire. Practice yoga. Cultivate oneself. Dream. Celebrate and appreciate. Share, give, and receive. Walk softly, live gently. Open up, expand, and include. Play. Take that walk now. I am focused, relaxed, and alert. I am confident. I am calm, cool, and collected under pressure. Calm. Breathe. Focus. Do not be afraid to perform. Pray. Enjoy. To love winning is easy; to love the battle requires toughness. I will not turn against myself in tough times. The crazier it gets, the more I will love it. During critical moments of execution, I focus my attention outside myself. Breathe, and breathe again. Smile lots. Be you, because everybody else is taken. Be aware. Create and envision. Forgive and accept. Enhance competencies and cultivate contentment. Be a friend. Be thankful. Revel in silence and nature. Surrender and trust. Expand, radiate, and dissolve. Simplify. I am enough.

Chapter Eight: Points to Ponder

1. Fun is the summit.
2. Fall awake with empowered mindfulness.
3. Pay attention to weak moments and make improved decisions.
4. Love and learn from failure. Fail your way to the top.
5. Be the person your dog thinks you are.
6. Continuously ask the two most important questions.

CHAPTER NINE

Playing Twister with Your Great-Grandchildren

Life is ten percent what happens and ninety percent how you react to it. I will not let living without an arm and a leg slow me down. I've learned to use it to my advantage. —Noah Galloway

Intention to Age 120

My late great-uncle Luther Warren lived till 106 years of age and kept his garden at his own house till the end. After his first wife Saretta passed, he married a young thing of 78. Uncle Luther was 95. He was considered a nut case in small town western Ohio in his era because he wasn't a meat and potatoes guy in the land of the family farmer. He was a lifelong thinker, learner, and doer. Evidently, he knew how to move well, eat well, and think well.

When you hear the words "setting goals" do you cringe, or are you energized by the idea of designing your circumstance? One of my favorite books is *Power of Focus* by Canfield, Hanson and Hewitt. The book has the most powerful and usable goal-setting technology I have ever used and I have been a devotee of goal setting for many decades. The authors help the reader discover their most meaningful short-term, mid-term, and long-term goals. That's how I decided to take my mountaineering addiction to the ultimate next level by climbing Everest for my 10-year mid-range goal back in the early 2000s. My longest term goal was elicited to be as follows: *I want to get on the floor and play with my great-grandchildren.* I have since added the Twister. Lots of grandparents can get on the floor and play with their grandchildren but I don't know many great grandparents who can muster the effort unless they have fallen and can't get up. The goal remains a compelling and memorable way for me to make ever improving health and wellness decisions throughout my remaining time on the planet.

It is highly doubtful you see a similar goal at age 50 if your life consists of being 60 pounds overweight, occupying a recliner all day, and refusing to give up your pack-a-day coffin nail habit. Chances are good you won't see age 60 unless drastic goals are set and achieved, but if you have been health conscience and you are of the mind to continuously improve, then set a similar target if the goal resonates with your soul.

With all said, I prefer "intention" to "goal." The word goal is a little stale after being a student of success philosophy since my early 20s. I love (or "lurve" as Steve Martin would say in the movie *All of Me*) the word intention.

Intention (n.) A thing intended; an aim or plan. The action or fact of intending.

The word feels powerful to me, hence the intention card vs. the goal card.

First things first, however. We need to talk about the big picture.

Your Big Idea

"Get the big idea, and all else follows," said B. J. Palmer.

Your big idea is your vision of your wellness future. Thinner, thicker, less anxiety, less negative stress, more fit, energetic, a home garden supplying all the veggies, sex three times a week, a 5K, a tenth marathon... or simply more energy after work to putter in the garden. Whatever your vision is, it is your intention and goes on your card.

Chapter Nine: Brain Train Exercise— Six Steps to Your Purpose

A. List ten personality traits you like about yourself. Example: your sense of humor, determination, desire to serve, etc.

1 _____ 6 _____

2 _____ 7 _____

3 _____ 8 _____

4 _____ 9 _____

5 _____ 10 _____

B. Select your three favorites.

1 _____

2 _____

3 _____

C. Referring to these favorites, make a list of five or more ways you enjoy expressing them. Examples: traveling, seeing patients, writing, teaching, fixing things, wiring homes.

1 _____

2 _____

3 _____

4 _____

5 _____

D. From this list select three favorites.

1 _____

2 _____

3 _____

E. Write a brief statement of your perfect world. Use the present tense. Describe what you want rather than what you don't.

_____

_____

_____

F. Put it together in one sentence with the following format: "The purpose of my life is to use my (insert your favorites from #2) by (insert your faves from #4) so that (insert your vision of an ideal world).

_____

_____

Example: the purpose of my life is to use my humor, courage, and curiosity by teaching, writing, and researching human behavior so that everyone is empowered to be, do, and have what they want.

I agree strongly with Dan Sullivan of The Strategic Coach who says "the next three years are always the most important period of your life." Do this additional exercise with me and dream of the cool possibilities.

A. Your present age. _____

B. Your age in three years. _____

C. How long do you think you will live? _____
   (Based on multitudes of clues from thousands of personal inputs).

D. Take a guess on how many extra years may be possible based on your new healthy Feet, Fork, and Fun lifestyle and your intentions.
   _____

E. Update your intention card and your purpose (if necessary) with short-term intentions: the next 1-3 months; mid-term intentions: the uber-important next 3 years; and long term intentions: 3 years to the rest of your life (includes, of course, your "extra" years from "D.")

F. Intentions should include the realms of physical (Feet, Fork, and Fun), relationships, financial, career, and personal.

G. With this much fun why not stretch yourself and envision living an active, exciting, Twister-playing life to 120 or beyond? Somebody has to do it, why not you and me?

The secret to living longer is to eat half, walk double, laugh triple, and love without measure.—Tibetan Proverb

Twister

Playing Twister with Your Great Grandchildren is an intention that will utilize all the technology and information I share in this book plus the inevitable refinements, research, and understanding that the future will inevitably provide.

Alas, many life events are beyond our control such as the fact that my son Kurt has his own life to lead and I am 56 years old. At this rate, even if Kurt starts a family tonight, I will be 96 years young playing Twister. Wow! That is exciting stuff and an adventure in the making.

How will I accomplish this? One step at a time, focusing on Food, Fork, and Fun daily and rebooting quickly when I screw up. Which I will but don't care as I will hit the reset button quickly, chuckle about it later, and flop on the floor with the future moppets. No kids? No problemo, you can raise children wherever you find them by volunteering in your favorite charities.

Never give up.—Anybody who ever did anything meaningful

Train Your Doctors (then outlive them)

There are health care providers and there are disease care providers. Both are necessary.

Health is defined by *Dorland's Medical Dictionary* as a "state of optimal physical, mental and social well-being, and not merely the absence of disease and infirmity." True health care providers are a small bunch and focus on the first half of the above definition: optimizing physical well-being. Practitioners reject the idea that a person is either sick or well and instead see the human being as being continually in flux along a continuum, then seek to optimize or improve the flux if you will.

Disease is defined by *Dorland's* as "any deviation from or interruption of the normal structure or function of any part, organ or system (or combination thereof) of the body that is manifested by a characteristic set of symptoms and signs whose etiology, pathology and prognosis may be known or unknown." Disease care, which is the vast majority of our "health" care system, essentially means treatment of a disease after it has made its appearance.

Since I am a basically healthy person except for some notably creaky joints, my plan is to use the Affordable Care Act's high deductible health insurance as catastrophic health care in case I get an expensive disease or accident. This is disease care insurance. For true health care or wellness care there generally is no health insurance coverage, so the object of the game is to live your life in a way that will maximize tone... hence the contents of this book.

In this regard, my personal health care "Team of Tone" (ha!) includes chiropractor, Dr. Dave Pilloni, who I see every week or two, and who has a foot in both camps (disease care when my spine and nervous system are misbehaving) and health care when I have a routine wellness adjustment. Matthew Smith, MD, also has a foot in both camps, and treats my creaky spine (disease care team) and also doubles as my tai chi teacher (health care team = tone). My disease care team includes my general practitioner (with occasional health care team attributes), orthopedic doc, and a dermatologist for once-a-year skin cancer screening. Special note: you may say, for example, isn't a preventative visit health care such as a yearly dermatological skin exam health care? Actually, no. Diagnosing a disease earlier (Read: skin cancer) is certainly advisable and smart but only activities designed to raise the vibration or tone of the human is true health, wellness, or tone. It's important to ponder and understand the similarities and differences between disease care, health care, and preventative care so (1) people get really clear on their responsibility of tone lifestyle choices and (2) our American society realizes the differences so we intelligently allocate resources in the future. Why? Our disease care system sure as shooting isn't working. Refer to Chapter Three, Have a Nice Decay.

No one much denies American health care is fracturing and imploding but the purpose of my discourse is to remind the reader and student of tone that it's all your responsibility. Maximizing the vibration of the body and mind that you inhabit is entirely on you. This should be freeing and empowering. Do you really want a government, bureaucracy, or any distracted health or disease care team of overworked (albeit dedicated) people overly focused on their sliver of focus or specialty while losing the big picture of a whole, complete Feet, Fork, Fun human being on the exam table?

Here is the point: You need an established team of people who know your philosophy of wellness. I think a GP whom you have educated to your minimalist philosophy in terms of medications, chemical exposure, and procedures and the chiropractor are the absolute minimum needed.

If you have reason to see a specialist, so be it, but you have to train them as well. Your providers of all stripes should be trusted advisors with you as benevolent dictator. Let them know that you are not going to take any medication, injection, procedure, test, or surgery until the CEO of tone (you) has established it to be absolutely necessary in consultation and research with your team, possibly including a second opinion. An exception would be an emergency situation where decisions need to be made whip fast.

Often, the best intervention is no intervention but trusting the body's wisdom or genetic potential to do its magic of sustaining life at a top level. Remember, your body is a highly tuned healing machine, especially now that you are ascending Mount Tone. If you look at your cardiologist and he or she is 50 years old, overweight, and shuffling down a hospital hall doing rounds while sucking oxygen from a tank and wearing a lab coat with a pack of cigs visible, run away fast. Far-fetched? Actual scenario from my local fish bowl.

Acupuncture, Chiropractic, and Massage Therapy: Yes, No, or Maybe?

The short answer is maybe, yes, and maybe. Incidentally each can be disease care, wellness care, or both. I have experienced all three professions often over the years and have referred many of my patients to the same. Although many people for thousands of years have found health with acupuncture it never seemed to work for me, even after repeated courses. With chiropractic care, my results were swift and lasting as a teen and now, at pushing 60, I continue to get adjusted weekly for the twofold benefits of maximizing brain health while minimizing nerve interference. I regularly see massage therapists but not because it feels good at the time—because it sure doesn't. A cruise ship fluff and buff massage is just that... fluff. I require a deep muscle fascia release technique that ranges from mildly uncomfortable to downright painful at times but minimizes my soft tissue accumulated stress and aids in muscular balance, circulation, and metabolic waste product removal.

Foam Rolling Was the New Stretching but P-Knotting Is the New Rolling

I was training hard for my second and ultimately successful climb of Denali (Alaska Range 20,320 feet and my second of the famed Seven Summits) when I ran my last mile. My calves were in significant spasm and pain which then caused me to limp which then aggravated my creaky chronic back. I started running at age twelve and at age forty-four I had to retire. What I didn't know at the time but have learned since was that if I self-tortured myself enough (called SMR, or self-myofascial release, essentially self-massage) with a foam roller, I probably could have continued to run. Today, part of my lifestyle is to foam roll with a four-foot foam roller (with six-inch diameter) before or after exercise and throughout each day with the P-Knot (www.P-Knot.com). I highly recommend every household to have a P-Knot and to go on their website and learn how to use it. Although painful at times and in spots, the more that these muscles and fascia soft tissue areas are "rolled," the less sore and irritating they are, and the more balanced the body becomes as it gets closer to its natural state. "Undo Your Day" is the P-Knot motto.

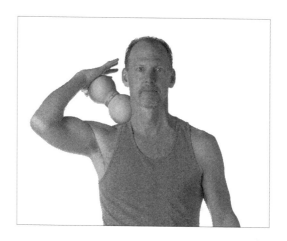

Even if I knew that tomorrow the world would go to pieces,
I would still plant my apple tree.—Martin Luther

90% Is the New 100%

Being perfect, or trying to be perfect, is a perfect disaster. Perfection is also a recipe for massive unnecessary negative stress and no fun. Stop it with that, dammit. Oh, that's right I do it myself. I am haranguing you because I'm reminding myself. I do battle with this habit on a daily occurrence. Be the best you can be using one-second living, philosophy, and practice and leave it there. It is what you do most of the time that counts, not all the time. Strive for kaizen or constant never ending improvement. Striving for perfection is perfect madness. Ninety percent attention is the new perfect. Ninety percent is the new one hundred percent. My suggested mantra: I am 100% 90% of the time.

"Take It Easy" is my favorite Eagles song and a pretty awesome mantra for one-second livers. (On the subject of livers, be nice to yours so you can continue being one.)

The Cure for Health Guilt

Remember my patient Kim from the book introduction? Kim was in her upper thirties, married with two kids, lived in a middle class home in a nice 'hood, had a good job, was a smart lady, and was miserable. The problem was that every time we talked in the adjusting room she told me how ashamed she was of her weight, as she yo-yo'ed between 30 and 50 pounds overweight no matter what she did, and the fact that she felt she was dropping the ball as a mom and wife. We talked endlessly in the office about exercise, nutrition, and how she could get the family involved, take the pressure off herself, lose the weight of the world she was carrying, have more fun, etc. She did indeed make some changes but never enough to make herself happy. I have to admit I wondered if she was serious enough or if I was getting the real story. Later she lost weight, a lot of weight, too much weight. She was diagnosed with an aggressive tumor and passed away quickly.

Kim passed when I was in practice for only a few years but I think of her situation often. We all inherently know that death is a part of life, but how very sad. How sad not just that she left her children without a mother, her husband without a wife, and her friends her, but how sad for her to have been needlessly miserable all those years. All those years she could have tweaked a few easy health hacks shared in this book and been lean, fit, and fun. For all anyone knows her cancer may have been prevented by living the active, non-inflammatory, and low stress lifestyle espoused within. The upshot is I have had Kim in mind on every page in this book.

People say that what we are all seeking is the meaning of life. I don't think that's true. I think what we are seeking is an experience of being alive.
—Joseph Campbell

Sly and the Family Tone

Parenting and marriage is often like climbing a difficult uphill, exhausting, circuitous, rocky trail with multiple false summits and an occasional great view. Too downer for you? You can have every intention in the world that your kids are going to eat acres of green things, never touch a Mountain Dew, and listen and obey every command from the bottomless well of wisdom liberally supplied by the sages of the living room. Remember I posited that 90% is the new 100% in personal health? Well, in parenting 75% is the new 100%. Do the best you can, strive daily to intend your family wellness goals, and ignore what you must... so your brain doesn't explode. Anyway, should it be any great surprise that your husband, wife, spouse equivalent, and children, and your dog for that matter, have different intentions than you?

If a problem arises on an airplane, parents are required to hook themselves up to oxygen first, then their children. Ideally, it should be identical to day-to-day family life. Too often, parents (often mom) see to everybody else's welfare before caring for themselves.

Parents preferentially placed on a pretend perfection pedestal to profess pfitness to the progeny. Sorry for that last sentence. What I'm saying is that the parental units (mom, pop, or parent equivalent) must take utmost care of themselves in exercise, nutrition, and headspace because the fam can't be well if mom and dad aren't well. You are most definitely NOT selfish for taking care of yourself. You, mom and/or dad, ARE selfish indeed if everybody gets cared for and you remain an unhealthy martyr.

What good is it to anyone if a parent drops dead of a heart attack at age 47? Martha was such a doting parent till she kicked the bucket and left the family devastated. Cardiovascular incidents, by the way, are more common in women than I ever expected. If the parents are unwell, their priorities are out of whack by spending every shred of time, money, and effort hovering over the screamers. Think that's you? Look in the mirror. What you see is bad parenting. Plus, as tone-d parents, you make an awesome role model for not only your kids, but the kids of your kids. What you do or don't do in your family today can resonate a hundred years down the road.

No family or kids? No problem. Once again, raise children wherever you find them. Can you be part of the solution in the community by volunteering in an organization that resonates? This is a tribe. Find your tribe or multiple tribes. This is how the world turns and how people stay vibrant and emotionally well. One of the biggest problems in especially older folks today is loneliness. Being introverted is fine but fight complacency, shyness, and habits that keep you away from people. Fake it till you make it and get out of any ridiculous comfort zones you may be in.

I'm Not Old, I'm Shabby Chic

Do you think you are too aged to reboot or too entrenched in old habits to make a quantum change in your life? Don't think you can Dyno even once let alone the five times per year recommended? There is simply nothing stronger than a made up mind. There is nothing more powerful than an idea that's time has come. Do you have one second? Do you want to be healthier? Use the STOP method then go. If your mind is made up to be well, then the hardest work is already done. Just do it and if you mess up put a huge smile on your face while you smack the do-over button.

What's Your Everest?

Just as your car was not designed to drive in neutral, your body and mind were not designed for checking out—otherwise known as retirement. First of all, minds and bodies only work well when used—just like a house that is vacant falls apart post haste. A grounded airplane becomes unflyable quickly. Show me a human addicted to TV and I'll show you a quickly deteriorating life potential. Have you heard that the average millionaire watches less than 5 hours weekly of TV while the average person on welfare watches north of 50 hours per week? Quick! Hit the reset button before rigor mortis hardens body and mind. Set your intentions, review them daily, and take action.

I have heard more than once that the average life span of a retired man is three years. The hypothesis being that the afflicted simply has no plan for spending time in retirement and the default apparently is death. Henry David Theroux said "people lead lives of quiet desperation"—

don't let it be you, brothers and sisters. Life is motion, intention, and action. Death is the opposite but let's put off that adventure as long as we can, shall we?

I never understood the mindset of people who say, "Oh, I would never want to live to 80, 90, or beyond." Why the hell not? Wouldn't you want to see what life is like then? We can't even imagine what cool technological advancements will be on the horizon. Sure, with time there will be heartache as friends and family will inevitably pass away. The way I see it our responsibility while here on earth is to do and be the best we can and to chase down and fulfill our purpose. I just want to look around and enjoy while on the journey.

You Used to Be a Star

Life originated from swirling gases in space made of star dust, later congealing into primordial ooze, then bacterial slime, followed by any team that beats the Red Sox, then pterodactyls, fluffy Golden Retriever puppies, and finally the crowning glory of them all... Usain Bolt. And it was good. I believe that the complexity of life could not have progressed, or even begun, without a swift kick in the butt from God to get the whole shebang started, but let's go back to the slime thing.

Bacteria are frenemies. Bugs are, in fact, way more friend than enemy. We exist rather nicely with a bajillion bugs inside and out. The goal of medicine in days past (though some still haven't gotten the change memo) was to wage war on bacteria. That understanding saved untold millions of lives but has had unforeseen negative ramifications.

The 4000-Year History of Medicine.

2000 BC "Here, eat this root."

1000 AD "That root is heathen! Here, say this prayer."

1865 AD "That prayer is superstition. Here, drink this potion."

1935 AD "That potion is snake oil! Here, swallow this pill."

1975 AD "That pill doesn't work! Here, take this antibiotic."

2000 AD "That antibiotic is poison! Here, eat this root."

The truth is we cannot survive without bacteria on us and especially inside us, so fighting bugs is a quixotic, unwinnable, and foolhardy endeavor but is exactly how mainstream medical care has "advanced" for the better part of the last two centuries.

The key to immunity is not to kill more bugs (bacteria) but to accentuate our genetic intelligence so our bodies, minds, and immunity remain as bulletproof as possible. Pathogens, or bad bugs, and out-of-control good bacteria can not kill and eat us for dinner IF our inborn genetic intelligence natural immunity is working on all 12 cylinders.

By striving for tone in body and mind we armor-clad our body's immune properties. In fact, how we live our lives is the only way to partner with our inborn intelligence. Striving to live the toned lifestyle is like walking arm in arm with the power that made the body. We cannot get healthier from an "outside in" pill, procedure, or surgery. We can only be well from "inside out" high vibrational tone. Traditional medical procedures are awesome at keeping us alive after a major car accident or disease but are simply not designed for keeping us healthy and our immune systems functioning like a twelve-cylinder Bugatti purring at redline.

What I am proposing is a partnership with your bugs. You are healthiest when you and your cooties are on the same team. Your health and wellness depend on it. In biology, it is called a symbiotic relationship: Both exist for the betterment of all.

What has proven a dismal failure is going to war with bugs. Using antibacterial sprays, soaps, and antibiotic pills in the long term have worsened our wellness because bugs adapt, become resistant, and get stronger. If the host human happens to be walking around and his/her resistance is down either from temporary or habitually poor lifestyle choices, the result is a weakened host and an available happy, healthy bug. If the bug happens to be a coronavirus (common cold) then you have a high chance of a cold. If the host human (you) is strolling around the world in a highly vibrational toned state, you could swap spit with the sickest person on the planet and you wouldn't get sick because your resistance (combo of genetic potential and tone) made your resistance bulletproof. The key is to get and stay toned. You have control of tone. You will never have control of the bugs around and within you. Likewise, you cannot control your God-given genetic potential. You only have control of how you live your life. Live it well and your internal innate strength and resistance will thrive and billions of naturally occurring hitchhiker germs will as well.

Health Futuring

The future of wellness looks only a little like today. Being the eternal optimist, I see a great deal of promise for the future but we have most definitely not arrived. It amazes me that grass-fed meat is so prevalent and that organic and home grown fruits and vegetables proliferate as much as they do. The seeds are there but the plant needs to mature.

The biggest change that will happen in the future is that people will accept once and for all that their health responsibility lies with them and not their mommy, daddy, doctor, the hospital, teacher, preacher, or God. I believe that the health insurance system will hasten this metamorphosis of understanding. Today's families getting majorly squeezed by insurance premiums certainly is a negative for nearly all families but because deductibles are so high it forces us to pay cash out of our pockets more and more rather than using an insurance card like a credit card that someone else is paying for. In the long run, people will be more inclined to take more responsibility for their health as traditional sickness care will be increasingly out of reach. We have a way to go for folks to take responsibility for themselves because in the news this past year was the advent of the sinister "affluenza" psychiatric disorder, defined as "a psychological malaise supposedly affecting wealthy young people, symptoms of which include a lack of motivation, feelings of guilt, and a sense of isolation." Affluenza was used as a defense in a recent high profile court case which I am sure something similar must have occurred just before the fall of the Roman Empire.

Second, in the coming world, drugs and surgery will be curtailed by a minimum of 50% within the next few years and most probably reduced to 10% or less from then on. It is killing us and disabling us. Surgeries, in the not-too-distant future, will be reduced significantly but not to the same percentage as drugs. Let's take a look at the lowly knee meniscus surgery. It's been done millions of times (including me twenty years ago) and many of them, according to today's research, were unnecessary. It seems these injuries would have healed in their own sweet time.

Imagine the marketing team meeting in Big Pharma when this went down: Hey team, profits are down to $50 billion, we have to come up with a new diagnosis pronto so we can pair a new combo of chemicals, test them on unsuspecting stooges, and drive profits through the ceiling where they belong. The result is a new drug I recently saw on TV for the newly created disease of internal clock loss in blind people. I don't wish to minimize the difficulties that blind people go through on a daily basis but a new drug for this seemingly made up condition, makes me laugh in a sinister slasher film kind of way.

Chapter Nine: Points to Ponder

1. Set your vision and intention.
2. Think two, three, or four generations down the road and raise children wherever you find them.
3. Train your doctors well.
4. Find and maintain your tribes.
5. Perfection reduces fun.
6. Live your future now.
7. Tone = natural immunity.

CHAPTER TEN

The Everest 70 Challenge

No one is born fit. Everyone who ever became fit did so through a thousand simple decisions -decisions they made every day to move, to purge imperfections, to eat the healthiest foods and to restructure their lives in pursuit of important goals.—Joe De Sena, founder of Spartan Race

The fishermen know that the sea is dangerous and the storm terrible, but they have never found these dangers sufficient reason for remaining ashore.—Vincent van Gogh

I didn't come this far to only come this far.—Unknown

We do not have to become heroes overnight. Just a step at a time.
—Eleanor Roosevelt

The sky is not the limit... I am.—T.F. Hodge

Adopt the pace of nature: her secret is patience.
—Ralph Waldo Emerson

In Chapter One, I shared the story of Catherine's average morning. I purposely didn't create her story to be over-the-top unhealthy, rather a common story shared by smart, busy families everywhere. Go back to the first few pages and jot down a few (or a dozen) simple doable ways that her family's wellness could improve. This will be a far better exercise than me harping at you more than I have already. My point is this: we all need to Dyno continuously and we all need to compete with the worthy adversary in the mirror, but first we need to identify what we are willing and unwilling to accomplish.

Compete With the Most Worthy Opponent: You

To challenge oneself is to be human. Humans compete. If not with others then certainly with themselves. The self is by far the greatest adversary.

The Everest 70 Challenge is a 70-day exercise in crushing your reset button. It's a big fat hairy Dyno. It may, in fact, be two or three of your five recommended yearly Dynos. We are not talking about tapping the button in a nambi pambi half-hearted manner but crushing it. Crushing the exercise reset button, crushing the nutritional reset button, and crushing the mindset button. In fact, squashing it till the wires pop out. Why the "Everest" in the Everest 70 Challenge? Because it is big, it is hairy, it is audacious, it's a huge challenge, it is dangerous, it is life changing, it is life enhancing, and it is a great metaphor for overcoming difficulties in our lives. The 70 refers to the days it takes to make an Everest climb and the number of days it takes to shift health habits into the awesome category. We are all climbing a Mount Everest. The wellness Everest! Every 70 days we should have a Dyno to maintain variety and motivation hence the five Dynos/year intention.

I want you to decide—it is as simple as that. Decide to be the best you that you can be. Decide once and for all to embrace your human potential. The past does not matter. Only the present and future matter.

Let's do this together, and remember it's fun to kick ass. This is about you only. How great will you feel about reaching your fitness, weight, and energy goals? Let me assure you that it is worth it. It feels (warning: overused adjective alert) AWESOME.

Kicking Your Own Ass: A Love Story

You don't even have to tell anybody that you are shaking up your tree of life. Let them see that wry smile of contentment on your face and wonder what the hell is going on. This is even more fun. If you want to tell your posse, go ahead, but choose carefully. Choose to tell only those who are unequivocally in your corner. Choose to share only with people who will root for you, not against you. If you do get the occasional hater or back stabber, "cancel" the comment in your mind and move on. You are winning and nothing will stop you on your pursuit of the holy grail of human potential.

I wonder how soon you will get your first compliment. I'll wager it will be sooner than you think. Very quickly your buds will wonder what you are keeping from them.

You are a role model, whether you know it or not—coworkers, friends, spouse, kids, strangers on the street, or on your Facebook page—everybody. Work the plan softly and proudly or loudly and proudly. Do which ever approach resonates with your soul and personality but just start. Start where you stand.

Challenge Basics

- I want you to fire, aim, and then get ready rather than ready, aim, and fire. In other words, start now where you are, where you stand. You are here now, so start here and now... and when I say "now," I mean this present moment because we have a moment, we have a second. Remember one-second wellness from the first chapter? Success is making a good decision in the moment. Make one now... to begin the challenge. Mark it down now in your calendar. Now mark down 70 days from now.

- There is nothing stronger than a made up mind. Nothing stronger than an idea that's time has come. Harness this power in yourself. Start.

- Get your E70C (Everest 70 Challenge) coaching and supplies or do it without any coaching or supplies except for your own resilience.

- In the last chapter we set some life intentions but for challenge purposes we will set some specific 70-day measurable goals. Set an "out there" intention Dyno or BHAG (Big Hairy Audacious Goal) for your wellness and your fun goals.

- Contact me for help at tim@drtimwarren.com.

In the Feet realm, measurable goals could be anything that is believable, realistic, and measurable in 70 days... but stretches your comfort muscles. It may include before and after weight, resting heart rate, blood pressure, body fat percentage, and body measurements.

Write down these starting numbers and goals in a special journal or on a dedicated page on your phone notes app. Make your Feet, Fork, and Fun lifestyle reality then test and document at 35 days and then again at 70 days. Take front and back pictures of yourself in the exact same skimpy bathing suit or the same pair of underwear. Guys: this doesn't mean you don't wash your u-trow for 35 or 70 days.

An example of goals might be to drop 20 pounds of fat and weigh 170 pounds with lowered blood pressure and heart rate with a body fat percentage of less than 30. Some folks talk to their doctors and get a blood test to measure markers of inflammation, that is certainly an option.

Chapter Ten: Brain Train Exercise

What's the difference between sickness, wellness, and fitness? In reality, they are different measures of a single quality: health. We can scientifically measure a number of components of health such as muscle mass, good and bad cholesterol, blood pressure, body fat, resting pulse, bone density, triglycerides, flexibility, respiration rate, etc. A blood pressure of 170/100 is considered pathological, 105/60 is consistent with a trained athlete, while a normal healthy or "well" BP would be 120/80, for example. A body fat of 40% is pathological, 10% would be fit, whereas 20% would be called normal or healthy. Therefore, everything you can measure about health exists on that old friend the continuum.

Sickness	Wellness	Fitness
170/100 BP	120/80 BP	105/60 BP
40% Body Fat	20%	10%

There are some health attributes that don't lend themselves to easy measurement, such as mental health, although depression is clearly mitigated by proper nutrition and exercise. The bottom line is fitness (the author's tone) provides a great margin of protection against the ravages of sickness and time—a super-wellness, if you will.

For your Fork or nutrition goals, try this on for size: A fistful of vegetables at each major meal, a hand-sized portion of good-quality protein at each mealtime. Remember the "My Paleosity Plate" diagram from Chapter Seven, Fork?

How about getting a freezer to purchase more meat from a grass-fed local herd? How about starting a container garden or adding to the garden outside this year? Have you tried growing sprouts for healthy salads all year long even in cold climes.

How about eating together as a family two additional days per week?

How about hosting a Paleosity potluck party once a month?

How about throwing out everything in your pantry that you know interferes with your health? Realizing that what one buys is usually what one consumes, how about the novel idea of NOT buying anything that is incompatible with a healthy body and mind? I know this one is a mind blower.

How about buying and decorating your very own personal water bottle and having it wherever you go?

How about instead of taking a sip of water you chug five big swallows each time?

How about packing healthy snacks for the work week in advance so you do not have to worry about it?

How about on Sunday shopping for everything and cooking in advance and freezing and refrigerating a week's worth?

As stated before, if you improve your physical, for example, your chemical and mental automatically ascend the continuum. Same with the other dimensions so don't put all your focus into one area and ignore the others. Go for the gusto—after all, it's your life.

Remember the biggest reason that people do not follow through with wellness is C.R.A.P.: complacency, rationalization, apathy, and procrastination. Are they figments of the past for you? I hope so. That, in and of itself, would be a home run, but most people have to do battle with those familiar villains daily. Don't despair. If it was easy, everybody would do it. If you have read this far, you are way ahead of the game. Keep putting one foot in front of the other.

When starting the Everest 70 Challenge, or for that matter anything else that may be new and scary, an additional foil often comes into play: the villain called "fear"—fear of making a change or the fear of the unknown. Remember the word neophobia?

FEAR: False Evidence Appearing Real

As a little kid, I was plagued with fear. I would not talk to adults or even to other kids until I felt comfortable, which seemed to take forever. I would not participate in any new activities with other kids because of fear, and it caused me much heartache. I was the painfully shy one with a death grip on mom and dad's leg. Then when I watched a horror movie with my older cousin, I would barely sleep for the following 2 months. I was scared to death. Later on, in junior high, I was scared to death of the girls. I was always scared of something. However, I innately knew that I was not serving myself so I decided to keep throwing myself out there on the world. I would be damned if I wasn't going to walk up to the plate and take my hacks.

At some point, imperceptibly slowly, I started learning from fears and failures instead of sprinting away from them. I realized that if you are not failing, you are not trying, and if you are not trying, you are not living. It took looking straight into the eyes of the dude in the mirror, warts and all, and deciding to do whatever I could do to improve myself. What about you? What do you need to say to the person in the mirror? What do you need to confront? We all have something. Do you have the brass balls or brass ovaries to confront and change?

In my teens, twenties, and thirties I failed at, among many other things, nearly flunking my sophomore year of college, nearly flunking out of grad school after a car accident caused a severe concussion, flunking my state boards the first go-around, getting fired from several jobs, in crushing debt several times, dropped out of the first triathlon I entered in the first hundred yards. Let me take a breath. I almost dropped a tree on my 5-year-old son's head.

I can barely cook, in fact, I have said in this book before I can barely boil water because I get confused with the ingredients. I have blown a couple of speeches in front of hundreds of people. I failed at a couple of side businesses and lost a ton of money. I failed at climbing many mountains the first time I tried. I failed in my first marriage and in multitudes of other relationships. I had to retire from a career that I loved, not because I wanted to but because my body had given up the ghost. I remember a spectacular fail decades ago when I did not speak to a beautiful young woman in a supermarket in Iowa who smiled at me in each aisle while I couldn't muster the testosterone to even say hello. One of my worst failures was having to tell my 8-year-old son that I was moving out of the house because his mom and I were getting divorced.

These are just a few of my failures, but I have grown from all of them. It's important to note that all these failures listed came during years of gradually losing the fear of failure (not that it ever completely leaves you). I stopped being as shy. Sure, every now and then I can regress a tad, but shyness and fear, I realized, didn't serve me. It wasn't part of my definition of Fun. In my school presentations I have given to thousands of children from grades two to college, one of my main tenets is "fail your way to the top." Everyone fails. We are supposed to fail in order to learn, adapt, and progress. We are supposed to fail in order to rise above, learn the lessons, and march forward with resilience. If you think you have not failed, (1) you have lived a meaningless life by not taking chances, (2) possibly you have failed but have not labeled it as such, or (3) you are a lying sack of you-know-what.

The big "aha" for me was realizing that I could not lose. Today, if I am pitching a media story, a proposal for a speaking engagement, or a book publisher, I realize I cannot walk out poorer than when I entered. I might get rejected, but I am going to learn a slew of things that will help me the next time around.

You are not Russell Crowe going into battle in *The Gladiator* where only one emerges alive. The worst manifestation of the self-imposed failure label is victim mentality.

Victimization is a fate almost worse than death because we give up control and default to whining. We no longer strive for success but spend that energy convincing ourselves and others why it is impossible to succeed or why the world is out to get us.

Since I described a large steaming pile of personal failures, I should add that I have a much, much longer list of amazing experiences, accomplishments, and friends made along the way. I wouldn't trade either list.

Back to the Challenge. Most 30-, 60-, or 90-day health challenges are standalone and in the scheme of things have little effect on long-term health habits becoming internalized even if they are effective in the short term. For example, *The Biggest Loser* is a popular TV reality show where people have lost a great deal of weight. Turns out only one of the "winners" has kept the weight off since the show and the others have actually gained the weight back PLUS more! I say right up front that tone can only be maintained with lifelong empowered mindfulness and work, but it doesn't mean that you have to dedicate your life to it. Remember that it's what you do most of the time that counts. With that said, challenges like the E70C can work.

Why do challenges work? Humans need focused, concrete, definable goals like quitting smoking within 6 months or finishing a Spartan Race on April 10th. How do you define steps while redrawing lifelong habits in exercise, nutrition, and mindset? The answer is the same way I climbed Mount Everest: one step at a time in the direction of my dreams. One changes his or her life one momentary wellness choice at a time with their intention firmly anchored.

Many toners appreciate a step-by-step graphic hand-holding so I have supplied a simple daily form (called the Week Sheet) that at a glance shows your progress. Download it for free at www.drtimwarren.com. If you need some one-on-one coaching, group coaching opportunities for your tribe or organization, or a speaker for your next rah-rah rally, see the above website for more details.

The possibility of a "post goal mortem" psychological letdown after the 70 days is eliminated by setting intentions for the next Dyno, even before we start.

Tone is an inside job. Health is within. Tone is an amalgamation of how a person lives their life in the Feet, Fork, and Fun dimensions modified by their unique genetic potential. None of my recommendations involve attempting to look like an airbrushed model, run a world record marathon, or become a Jedi knight. It's all about tiny daily wins and improvements that foster self-satisfaction and facilitate further incremental wins.

Will you turn the metaphorical next page of your life to begin? Will you step up to bat... even if it's Nolan Ryan pitching? Will you climb your

Everest? Will you feel the fear and do it anyway? I certainly hope so because at the very least you will have great tales to tell indeed.

What do I need this moment? What will serve me best right now? Remember that attempting something this moment to enhance your time on earth is worth all the treasure in Moria.

Chapter Ten: Points to Ponder

1. Self Challenge = Self Improvement = Self Respect = Self Love.

2. Fire, Aim, Ready!

3. Constantly stretch your comfort muscles.

4. Tone = Super Wellness.

5. Climb your own Mount Everest not anybody else's.

6. Many invest in stocks or bonds, not as many invest in body and mind.

Extra Cool Stuff,
otherwise known as the Appendix

Chapter One

Another way to explain the concept of tone is with vibration.
A high vibrational human being (read: toned) eats high vibrational food, broccoli for example, versus a low vibrational food, such as a chocolate cream donut.

A high vibrational person does high vibrational activities such as taking the stairs at work, versus a low vibrational activity like taking the elevator habitually.

The high vibrational human embraces learning and experience and listens to an audiobook in the car while going to work versus low vibrational brain use such as mindless commercial-laden junk radio.

Tone is the mission of wellness acolytes who embrace Feet, Fork, and Fun. It's like summiting Everest and safely returning to base camp... every day. Tone is the health equivalent to actor Cuba Gooding's all-encompassing word "quan" in the movie *Jerry Maguire*.

Chapter Two

Have you ever thought about what happens when you get a little cut in your finger? Somehow your body knows instantly where the break in the skin is and sends white blood cells to fight any chance of infection. Then more substances and chemicals are produced to stem blood flow, form a clot, then a scab, which eventually catches on your sweater and flies off to reveal... brand new skin. The body miraculously repaired itself and you didn't even tell it to or even buy the regrow body parts app. Imagine if your automobile could self-heal? One day at Dave's Market, a runaway grocery cart dents and scrapes the side of your car. Not to worry, the next day a scab has formed and a couple of days later falls off to reveal brand new smooth-as-a-babies-behind yellow paint on your '62 Corvair. Sadly enough, most of us do not appreciate the wondrous inner miracles that our bodies perform millions of times a day. One does great honor to our genetic potential by living a balanced, energized, exciting life with the prerequisite attention spent to the three dimensions of life: physical, chemical, and emotional or Feet, Fork, and Fun.

The human body, even though it self-heals and self-regulates miraculously, can be overwhelmed and interfered with (poor health habits and vertebral subluxation, for example); hence the propensity for disease and dysfunction among young and old today. The point and purpose of this book is to reveal how minimizing lifestyle interferences to the body's self-healing while simultaneously eliminating the overwhelm that stymies people's progress.

Hippocrates said, "All living creatures are either growing or dying." What he meant was humans are dynamic and continually involved with balancing the opposing constructive and destructive biological processes. Constructive processes promote bodily repair, regulation, balance, homeostasis, and tone. Destructive processes include accumulating negative stresses in the physical realm (sitting too much with a phone lodged in your neck), chemical realm (eating fried food daily), or emotional dimension (you just got fired). If these accumulating negatives are above the body's ability to adapt then health spirals downward. To summarize, life is different each moment of existence. In each instant we either move toward health and life or toward disease and death. Your choice.

Three necessities for a maximized healthy life.

1. A daily intentional focus toward purity, wellness, health, and life.

2. A lifestyle that sufficiently supplies body and mind everything it needs to function, heal, and grow.

3. A healthy nervous system free of interference.

Chapter Three

I casually mention in the first two pages of this chapter that everybody who owns a spine should see a chiropractor for "brain exercise." Many think that chiropractic care is only for back pain, neck pain, headaches, or tsutsugamushi disease but I think the biggest positive of chiro care is a brain–body reset to homeostatic balance, closer to the perfection of our design. In my opinion the best part of chiropractic care (again only for anyone and everyone who own a spine) is a minimization of lifestyle-induced interference (we doctors of chiropractic call this subluxation) that restores the natural brain–body connection. In short, brain exercise.

However, most go to the chiropractor for natural pain relief so dig into this cool stuff from www.palmer.edu/gallup-report/sources/. In a nutshell summary: chiropractic is safe, they are real doctors based on training, it works, many people go (over 50% of U.S. adults), and chiropractic care helps back and neck pain

How do you get a good chiropractor if you don't already have one? It sometimes reveals a conundrum as some chiropractors are more interested in either the pain relief or treatment of disease type care and others are more of the global, holistic, brain exercise type folks. My advice is do your research, remembering that you are the CEO of you. Check out the websites I share here for background education then start polling. One of the best strategies to find the right DC for you and your family is to poll your friends, family, and acquaintances and ask them who they go to. Try to get a minimum of three recommendations before you decide and then focus your research on the doctor's website. At this point call the office and ask questions. You should feel a warm fuzzy deep down about the doctor and office before you step foot in the front door.

Resources:

International Chiropractors Association   www.chiropractic.org

American Chiropractic Association   www.acatoday.org

Special Note: Dr. John Manning is a chiropractor with a specialty of Applied Kinesiology. I see him periodicaly to screen endocrine (hormonal), immune, digestive, and cell detoxification pathways. See www.icak-usa.com or call Dr. Jay at 508-835-8800.

Chapter Four

Confused about good vs. bad stress? Here are some examples of the baaaad.

Seven negative Feet stresses: being born, carrying a child on one side, car accidents, sitting in the bleachers at kids' games, sleeping on a plane, doing sit-ups.

Seven negative Fork stresses: handling pressure-treated wood without gloves, eating fast food, breathing the air in Kathmandu, ingesting preservatives and chemicals, more than two alcoholic drinks, eating fried food, drinking water in Flint, Michigan.

Seven negative Fun stresses: getting angry, watching the Red Sox, dealing with pushy sales people, snakes on a plane, too much debt, frustration, not getting homework done.

Chapters Five and Six

FAQ #6: "Can you write me a prescription for medical marijuana?" A: What the hell? No. But I would personally take a vaporizer dose with a higher cannabinoid concentration relative to THC way before I would take an ibuprofen (Advil) and absolutely before any acetaminophen (Tylenol) or opioid product. The vape is less injurious to delicate body tissues than smoking. Smoking anything is horrible regardless of the substance.

Some related Feet websites that rock:

www.p-knot.com for awesome self-massage and self-healing.

www.bodybuilding.com for routines and gym workouts.

www.yoga.com

I would love to recommend a functional training site but there is simply too much information out there so Google away and apply what resonates.

Chapter Seven

Just so you get the Paleosity big idea, enjoy several recipes from Dr. David Pilloni, my chiropractor in Warwick, RI (401-738-6477).

Sweet and Spicy Bacon Brussel Sprouts

Ingredients:

1 pound brussel sprouts, cut stem and quarter

8 bacon strips uncured, diced

2 tablespoons honey

Sriracha sauce to taste

Directions:

1. Preheat to 350 degrees.
2. Fry diced bacon in large pan on stovetop.
3. Add brussel sprouts and saute for about 5 minutes.
4. Add garlic, honey, and sriracha, stir to combine.
5. Pour contents into glass baking dish and bake 30 minutes or until golden brown on top.
6. Enjoy!

Crockpot Paleo Beef and Broccoli

Ingredients:

1 1/2 lbs flank steak or skirt steak cut in thin strips against the grain

1/3 cup arrowroot powder

2 tablespoons avocado or olive oil

3 garlic cloves finely chopped

1/2 cup coconut aminos

1/4 cup water

1/4 cup honey

1 tablespoon sriracha

1 small onion finely chopped

2-3 broccoli crowns cut into florets

Directions:

1. Mix the steak and arrowroot powder in the crockpot until evenly coated.

2. Whisk remaining ingredients, except onion and broccoli, and pour over steak.

3. Add onion.

4. Cook on low for 4-5 hours or on high for 2-3 hours. During the last 1/2 hour, add broccoli and stir.

5. Enjoy!

Avocado Egg Boats

Ingredients:

2 avocados sliced in half, pits removed

4 large eggs

8 strips uncured bacon

Pinch of sea salt

Pinch of black pepper

Pinch of garlic powder

Directions:

1. Place avocado halves in large muffin pan holes to create an "avocado boat."

2. Season each avocado boat with salt, pepper, and garlic powder.

3. Crack one egg into each boat.

4. Bake boats in oven on 350 degrees until eggs are cooked to liking.

5. While avocado boats are baking, fry bacon and place 2 strips over each boat.

6. Enjoy, that's an order.

Book suggestion: *The Paleo Solution: The Original Human Diet*, by Robb Wolf.

Chapter Eight

To survive the ascent and descent on Mount Everest in 2008 I had a secret weapon. A wadded single sheet of paper in the outside pocket of my one-piece down suit. My plan was if I was on my last legs of survival at 29,000 feet, I would review my chicken scratch and survive. Affirmations are powerful success stimulators. My affirmations on that scrap of paper still resonate with me. Take a gander at mine and create your own by downloading a copy of the actual paper. Go to www.drtimwarren.com.

Chapter Nine

www.hasbro.com/twister

Chapter Ten

Because you purchased this book you qualify for a free coaching session with Dr. Tim. See the website for details and don't forget to Dyno the Everest 70 Challenge easily with the Feet, Fork, and Fun "Week Sheet," also available free on www.drtimwarren.com.

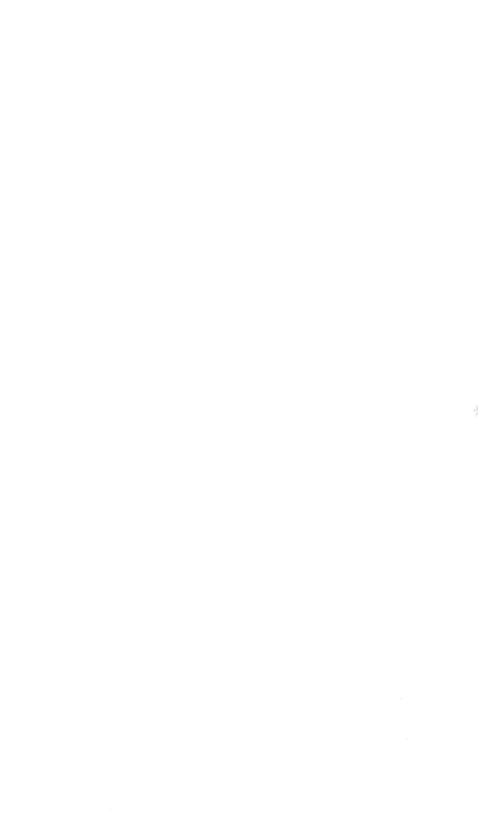

40788483R00099

Made in the USA
Middletown, DE
22 February 2017